A True Story c

Still Wearing My Heels

Surviving SJS/TEN:

The Cruelest Syndrome of Modern Medicine

Michelle Frazzetto

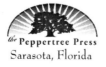

the Peppertree Press
Sarasota, Florida

The scriptures used in this edition are quoted from
The Holy Bible, New International Version®, NIV®,
Copyright© 1973, 1978, 1984, 2011, by Biblica, Inc.®,
and *The Holy Bible, Revised Standard Version*®, RSV®, Copyright© 1952.
Used by permission. All rights reserved worldwide.

Copyright © Michelle Frazzetto, 2014
All rights reserved. Published by the Peppertree Press, LLC.
the Peppertree Press and associated logos are trademarks of
the Peppertree Press, LLC.
No part of this publication may be reproduced, stored in a
retrieval system, transmitted in any form or by any means, electronic,
mechanical, photocopying, recording, or otherwise, without prior
written permission of the publisher and author.
Graphic design by Rebecca Barbier.

For information regarding permission,
call 941-922-2662 or contact us at our website:
www.peppertreepublishing.com or write to:
the Peppertree Press, LLC.
Attention: Publisher
1269 First Street, Suite 7
Sarasota, Florida 34236

ISBN: 978-1-61493-288-8
Library of Congress Number: 2014913684
Printed in the U.S.A.
Printed October 2014

For we walk by faith, not by sight.

2 CORINTHIANS 5:7 (RSV)

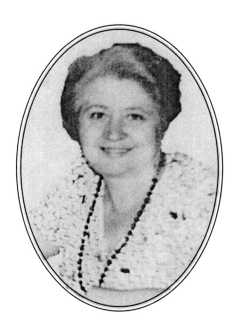

In Honor of My Mother

Without whose never-ending love,
unwavering strength, infinite patience,
and unfaltering faith, this book
would not have been written.

Mom, I love you.

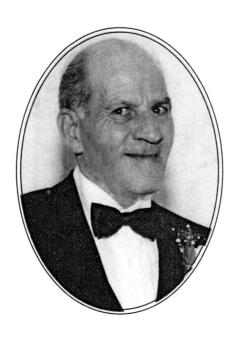

In Loving Memory of My Dad

*Papa, it pains me that you aren't here
to see me achieve this. Thank you for
being the greatest father any daughter
could want. You're always in my heart
and I love you.*

Author's Note

Dear readers, three years ago I embarked on a profound journey writing this memoir without eyesight. Family, friends, and acquaintances inspired me to share my story with you, hoping I would educate and reveal to society what can happen when a person has an extreme reaction to a prescription medicine. My greatest wish is to help raise awareness of this syndrome and perhaps save your life or the life of someone you know. Reliving my tragedy was emotionally painful for both my mother and me but she remained by my side encouraging me to tell it completely and fearlessly. To the best of our abilities we have recalled the medical terminology, the experiences, the conversations, and actual scenarios. Warning: the medical photos may appear graphic. Some of the names, places, and medical-care facilities mentioned in this book have been changed.

Michelle Frazzetto

June 2014

Editor's Preface
Working with a Blind Writer on a Classic Hero's Journey

by Denege Patterson

Michelle doesn't think of herself as a hero, but I believe she is. Without eyesight and disfigured by a horrible reaction to a simple medication, she reclaimed her life and was still wearing her heels when I met her three years ago. Michelle's friends and acquaintances had encouraged her to write a book about her experience with SJS/TEN, but how could she write a book? She was blind.

A friend of Michelle's saw an interesting book review in the local newspaper. It was the life story of an artist in her nineties whose mother and father had once been the caretakers for Thomas Edison. The book was *Edisonia Native Girl.* Michelle called the reporter for the name of the writer. When Michelle contacted me in 2011 to assist with her memoir, I was helping the artist provide speaking programs, book signings, and an art show at the Edison Estate.

As a busy volunteer I didn't think I could take on another project. But when Michelle told me about her desperate struggle to survive SJS/TEN and recapture her vibrant life, I was intrigued. I recognized her passion, spunky survival, and her great sense of humor. In my former career I had been a pastoral counselor and marriage and family therapist. After retirement I retained my lifelong interest in working with people as they embarked on a hero's journey. I didn't know anything about working with the blind but I certainly wanted to learn. I said, "I'm interested, but I have to think about this. This is not something I normally do; I write academic nonfiction and I'm not sure if I should take on another project right now. I would like to meet with you before I decide. Either way I can't start today; you would be number nine on the list. Could you give me a few weeks? I will call you."

Did I say a few weeks? Michelle waited on tenterhooks for two months. I reassured her, "My schedule is better now and I would like to meet with you. Would it be possible for you to come to the Indian Mounds at Pineland where I am a tour guide, and may I offer you my first tour for the blind?" (The Randell Research Center at Pineland, a relatively new program of the Florida Museum of Natural History, had not yet established an official tour for the blind. I was glad to make one up for this occasion.)

"Yes, of course," said the gracious and beautiful Michelle. "My friend Karen will accompany me." When I recommended wearing sneakers on the Calusa Heritage Trail, Michelle commented, "Okay, I'll try to find a pair. Normally, I always wear high heels." I wondered to myself: *how can a blind person walk in high heels*?

We met; the short tour went well. Michelle could feel the sun and the wind on her face, hear the birds, sense movement in the trees, feel the crunch of gravel on the path, and distinguish the changes in the elevation of each mound as Karen guided her along. My book was in the gift shop. Michelle held it in her hands, praising how it felt. When it came time to discuss Michelle's book I told them the truth, "Michelle, I would like to work with you, but I have some conditions."

Michelle answered hesitantly, "Okay, but are you sure you are willing to take me on?"

Yes. I was under the impression she was literate, intelligent, and capable of writing her memoir with just a little editing help from me. She was of the opinion I would record her words and type them.

I said, "Can you type up something and send it to me by email?"

Michelle stopped cold, speechless, thinking to herself, *is this lady crazy? I'm blind.* But she was her mother's daughter, courteous and obliging, and she said nothing. She didn't have to; I saw her expression. I explained, "Because after knowing all you went through, I don't think I could capture the emotions like you could. I believe you have it in you and it is ready to come out. If you can type, I can edit. I think you can do it."

I paused… Karen winked; I was on the right track. Michelle seemed a little insecure. She spoke tentatively, "Well my spelling and grammatical ability won't be the best. I haven't seen words in twenty-five years."

I said, "I will help you with that."

Michelle continued, "But I'm not sure about my computer. My computer is old, and it may not be compatible to yours."

I asked, "Does someone help you with the computer?"

"Yes, I have a computer teacher."

"Then we will figure it out."

Silence. Now I was the one on tenterhooks. I truly believed her story would be best if she wrote it. I could never capture the experience as well as Michelle could. She was articulate and expressive, friendly, outgoing, emotional, and passionate about life. I asked her to blurt straight from the heart and I would edit it to make it easier on the reader's eyes but not make any substantial changes. It would be her book alone. A wry smile came over her face. Or maybe it was a grimace. Karen beamed at me.

I repeated the question, "So can you type?"

She admitted, "Well, yes, I can type. I was an administrative assistant. My electronic reader, JAWS® reads it back to me."

I persisted, "So would you be willing to write the book and let me edit it?"

"I guess so," she agreed, rather half-heartedly. On the way home in the car with her dear friend Karen, Michelle confessed that she didn't think she could do this. "With those *conditions*, how the heck am I going to write my own book? I'm blind, for God's sake! I go to the doctor every other day. I can't write a book!"

Karen said rather bravely, "Well, if you want *her* to help, I guess you're just going to *have* to do it!" Years later, after getting to know one another, all three of us recount this sequence today with great laughter.

Michelle proved she could follow through. She contacted her computer teacher to find out how to send her writings as an attachment. When it all seemed possible, she wrote her first email to me, "Thank you for making one of my dreams come true!! It means so very much to me!!"

I was pleasantly surprised when Michelle sent me Chapter One. It captured my interest immediately and held my attention to the end. It was a great start. By email I told her so, and offered to make a copy, keeping the original intact by editing only the copy, increasing the font and spacing to make her words easy for the reader to see, inserting punctuation, and finding just the right word. Michelle responded, "You are such an angel!!! I didn't want to put too much burden on you, but if you really don't mind editing it, I would greatly appreciate it!! Learning the Word program, and using JAWS® commands when working in Word is already going to be a great challenge."

I replied, "You can take your time. I understand that it is a skill like playing the piano. I'm not in any rush."

She wrote, "I'm not in any rush either."

I concluded, "Good! Because it took me nine years to learn how to play the piano."

Thus began a most remarkable three-year journey. The next experiment was to discover how she was going to perceive the edits so that she could approve or reject them. I couldn't use the old editors' tricks of writing notations in the margins or using strike-throughs and replacements; she couldn't see them and her electronic reader wouldn't read them properly. I couldn't even use the new, electronic editors' tricks such as redlining, double-underlining, boldface, and markups. JAWS® would read both the old and the new with no distinction between them. JAWS® could not tell different colored text, or italics from non-italics, or different fonts. We had to devise a creative new way to edit. We decided I would send an edited copy, and Michelle would listen and determine whether she liked the sound of the edit. She would just have to trust the spelling, punctuation, and paragraphing. If she liked the sound, we would proceed to the next chapter. If she disagreed with the sound, we would re-edit the chapter together on the phone.

Our telephone editing procedure was simple. Michelle

listened to the edited text using a hand-held recorder to state a unique "key word" that appeared near any phrase she wanted to edit. She could make any number of changes throughout the chapter. Later, while I was on the phone with Michelle, I would do a computerized "word search" for her key word, find the spot, and listen as she recited to me what she wanted it to say. I would use earphones and take dictation as she spoke. Although she had a flawless auditory memory of all previous versions and could pick and choose which version was most to her liking, she had to trust my editor's eye for how it appeared to the reader's eye. *What an incredible amount of trust is required from a blind author working with a sighted editor!*

All the drafts would be dated and stored in my computer. Michelle's computer would have her original version and the current version, and eventually the final version. She sent completed chapters to her sister's computer as a backup.

With the editing procedures established we developed a routine. Michelle reached deep into her soul to write her story—or should I say "allegory"—as this was a classic hero's journey. For me the editing process became second nature as her deep story emerged. I couldn't wait for the next chapter.

Her first few chapters drew me into her late teens and early twenties. I was captivated by the experiences of a sighted, innocent young girl. Her graduation trip to Italy was a great example. I felt happy for her, as her own parents must have. I witnessed a deep courage as she faced her first job interview in Manhattan wearing her sassy high heels. I was touched by her conflicting loyalty to a girlfriend applying for the same job. The inner therapist in me noticed how during her young years she remained true to herself as she overcame each difficult challenge. She established herself as a functioning member of society and perhaps a future head of a family. I felt such hope for her.

Just when her life had seemed perfect, BLAM! She was prescribed a medication that sent her over the threshold into the unknown, fighting for her life. I never read or edited so fast in my life! I wanted to see what was coming next. As a mother, I admired how Michelle's mother's love revealed itself. Her mentors, helpers, and a number of believers multiplied her sacred context, a true example of faith in action. I felt uplifted.

Michelle began to send parts of a chapter recounting how at the edge of a miserable abyss, she faced a choice between life and death. Reliving this part of her journey while writing this book, she entered a Dark Night of the Soul. She had been through it before and never wanted to go through it again, yet, here it was, for all the world to see. She didn't know if she could continue. I waited. I knew from the classic hero's journey and from my experience as a retired pastoral counselor that a spiritual crisis when combined with Michelle's own faith had the power to transform her life—if she would let it. This part was not easy for her. We talked, cried, and laughed together. Michelle's mother stood by her, confirming her ability to continue. Michelle came up with the idea of inserting relevant scriptures in the beginning of each chapter. As she reconnected with her faith in the context of writing this book, an amazing strength came from deep within her soul.

This is the universal appeal of her book. All of us at one time or another in our lives must face our trial by fire. We need to reach out to a power greater than ourselves, rise up from the ashes, and find ourselves transformed into something more than we otherwise could ever be.

"I couldn't have written this book five years ago," she said, "the timing had to be right."

For me, it was a monumental privilege to work with this heroic young woman. May you find inspiration and strength as you accompany her on her hero's journey.

Denege Patterson, Editor

Bokeelia, FL
June 2014

Doctor's Foreword #1

Michelle is lucky to be alive. When she first came to my office she had already recovered from TEN, or "toxic epidermal necrolysis" literally "poisonous death process of the skin." She suffered from blindness, disfigurement, and chronic conditions due to a severe reaction to a prescribed medication. The TEN Syndrome is extremely rare but it can happen across a range of patients taking all kinds of medications, and it causes death in 25-35% of cases. Although patients have a very small chance of contracting TEN, this life-threatening condition is always considered a medical emergency.

Typical clinical signs of TEN initially include areas of discoloration of the skin with involvement of the mucous membranes especially the eyes, followed within minutes to hours by the onset of epidermal detachment characterized by the development of blisters. The surface area of the detachment of the skin is the main discriminating factor in distinguishing severity between the less deadly Stevens-Johnson Syndrome and TEN, with TEN the most severe. Management in the acute stage involves prompt identification and withdrawal of the culprit drug(s), rapidly initiating supportive care in an intensive care unit. A multicenter study conducted in the USA showed that the survival rate was significantly higher in patients who were transferred to a burn unit within seven days.

When Michelle came into my office she was involved in the more chronic aftermath of TEN including blindness, pain, scarring of the skin, shortness of breath, difficulty eating, and the permanent destruction of all the mucous membranes of the body. Due to combined involvements she needed inter-disciplinary support such as the services of an ophthalmologist as well as specific treatments to aid her other sensory and internal organs.

My staff and I have the utmost respect for Michelle. She is a living example of faith, hope, and perseverance in the face of unimaginable difficulties. We know that this book will be a source of inspiration to all readers.

Richard Torricelli, MD

Fort Myers, Florida
June 2014

DOCTOR'S FOREWORD #2

This is a moving story of many things: the healing power of a mother's unflagging determination, the miraculous power of faith and prayer, the courage and persistence of a heroic young woman's indomitable spirit, and the healing power of love—God's love, a family's love, the love of a dedicated group of doctors and nurses who stayed by Michelle amidst the incompetence, insensitivity, and arrogance that manifests itself all too often in healthcare today; and ultimately, a triumphant love of life that rose above betrayal and abandonment to find a deeper vision, even in the throes of blindness.

It is also a story of lessons. Today in the West we have arguably the most technically advanced medical science known to humanity—particularly when it comes to crisis intervention—and yet our vision of what it means to heal is still very much clouded by a materialist reductionism that treats primarily symptoms without regard to underlying physiology, that is still inhibited by an ethos of "dispassionate objectivity" that misses the big picture of what it means to be human, and which cries out to us to reconnect with a more authentic, soul-based, individualized medicine, that goes beyond the pharmaceutical algorithm into deeper reliance upon true thinking, heart-based feeling, and practically developed intuition. Michelle's story is a reminder to us all of how far we've yet to go.

Dr. Robert Kellum, ND, PhD, L.Ac.

Portland, Oregon

June 2014

AUTHOR'S INTRODUCTION

I agonized for weeks over my relationship with David. I loved him so much I didn't want anything to change between us. I was no longer the vibrant, self-assured young woman he had met two years prior. I was now in a wheelchair unable to walk. I was blind and disfigured; my long, beautiful blonde hair was gone. I was a mere fraction of the person that I once was on the outside. My heart and fiery spirit remained the same but I didn't know if that was enough for him to stay true to his promises. He had already gone through three months of emotional suffering as I lay in a coma fighting for my life. So much had been taken away from me, all I had left to give was an inner strength and the profound love I had for him. Physically the pain was unbearable; emotionally I was distraught. I did not know how I was going to rise above the complete devastation, and how I was going to live through this life-altering tragedy.

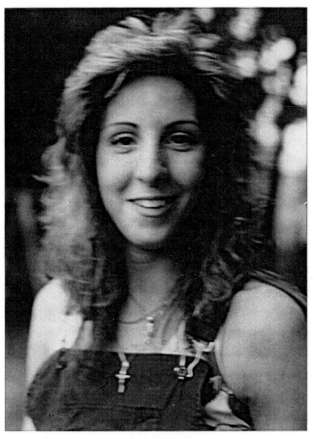

Michelle before the Accident

May the God of hope fill you with all joy and peace
as you trust in him...

—ROMANS 15:13

CHAPTER ONE

I was seventeen years old and still in my cap and gown when my girlfriends and I decided we should take the summer off. Why not celebrate our freedom, go to the beach, travel, get fun jobs, and live life to the fullest?

As a graduation gift I was given a ticket to Italy. My trip was absolutely enchanting. My sister Teresa and her husband resided in a villa on lands surrounding a king's summer palace near Torino. Together we visited medieval castles and walked past vineyards. We ate at trattorias, savoring home-made Italian dishes in courtyards beneath garden trellises. I sampled my first glass of wine, delizioso. Teresa's in-laws offered their villa on the Italian Riviera where I spent my days basking in the sun and watching the spectacular sunsets over the Ligurian Sea.

I made some lasting friendships in Italy. Imagine a young girl my age meeting Italian guys. I met Attilio and Alex at their uncle's hair salon. They were both incredibly handsome, each in a different way: Attilio had an exquisitely defined face with smiling eyes, and Alex was rugged-looking with chiseled features. I was extremely attracted to Attilio, yet his younger brother, Alex, had a serious crush on me. Our group would go to tiny cafés to enjoy a cappuccino together. In Italy it is very popular to go for a passagiata in centro, a walk through the center of the city, passing fountains and statues, and exploring little boutiques and shops down cobblestone alleys. We strolled through the Parco del Valentino along the Po River, with benches, little round tables and chairs, and beautiful gardens.

Theresa introduced me to Sonia, a girl close to my age. Sonia was an only child and in her spare time she worked in her parents' pizzeria. When it was busy I gladly helped; it was always so much fun. Sonia's parents had a villa in Lucca in the region of Toscana south of Turin. Through Sonia I met Roberta, a friend who lived in Lucca. During my stay there, we drove to the leaning *Torre di Pisa*. We went to concerts together, and on the endless sunny days we wore our bikinis to the beach where we would flirt with the young, romantic Italian guys. We also took long, leisurely road trips to France and Monaco.

Theresa and her husband Guido took me to Venice—my first ride on a gondola—simply romantic. (I had thoughts about the good-looking gondolier.) The city was steeped in history, legends, and beautiful architecture. I was most fascinated by the *Ponte dei Sospiri di Venezia,* Bridge of Sighs, connecting the interrogation rooms of the Venetian Doge's Palace with a prison across the canal. Upon this bridge the convicts would sigh, knowing it would be the last time they saw Venice on their way to confinement, never to see daylight again. (Little did I know this was a premonition of my future.)

It would be a summer I would always remember. On the plane coming back to New York I wondered about my new life ahead. Although the romantic part of me would have loved to follow in my sister's footsteps marrying a wonderful Italian man and moving to Italy, I instinctively knew that my immediate future existed in those high-rise office buildings across the river in Manhattan.

I couldn't wait to come home and tell Christine about my summer. She had been a friend since fourth grade, always at my house, and my constant companion. She lived with her parents on Staten Island, the youngest of three including Joanne and Johnny. At the age of nine I had a secret crush on Johnny. He always treated me like a little sister. He was someone I could look up to. As teenagers Christine and I went to different places to see him play guitar in a band. These occasions were rare since I was not allowed to "hang out" or date until age eighteen.

Christine and I had decided before leaving on my trip to seriously start looking for a job in September when I turned eighteen. We both felt excitement and apprehension about going into New York City to apply for our very first jobs. This would be the first time going into the city by ourselves. The thought was daunting. We didn't know what to expect or how to dress for it; we weren't even sure we could walk in high heels.

Christine provided moral support and encouragement for me as I did for her. We were mutually delighted when the employment agency scheduled us both for an interview at an investment company. I excelled in math; my typing and shorthand skills were outstanding. We waited three weeks before the human resources department phoned to offer me the job. I hesitated, thinking of Christine. It was the first time I was asked to choose myself over a friend. I discussed it with Christine and she supported me. She was confident another opening would become available. Feeling reassured, I accepted the position. I could never have imagined how this ordinary decision would alter the whole journey of my life.

It was an incredible first year; I had much to learn. The transition from being a young girl just out of high school to being a Wall Street Yuppie overwhelmed me. I was immediately inundated in the position of personal secretary for the manager and assistant manager, as well as secretary for twelve other people including accountants and payroll clerks. Jill was my assistant manager. Jill and I lunched together and sometimes went out on weekends, developing a good friendship. For eleven months we worked together smoothly; then she was promoted to a new department next door. I felt both happy for her, and personally sad to be losing her as my assistant manager. She was a mentor and a friend.

A young man named David was hired to replace Jill. I was unprepared for the difference between David and Jill's management style, and how their presence or absence changed my professional life. He seemed to be a breath of fresh air for everyone in the department except me; I wasn't quite sure why. He was a handsome young executive who looked great in a business suit. He joined the company with a lot of new ideas. His charm captivated the office women especially Jill. He had beautiful blue eyes and a kind, patient, and gentle demeanor. The men in the department respected his ability to be fair and down-to-earth. He just didn't impress me. When I learned that I was going to be his personal secretary I felt very uneasy. For some reason we clashed. We hardly ever saw eye-to-eye. The letters that I composed never pleased him. The reports that I typed up never went his way. It caused me a lot of aggravation. I actually hated going to work every day knowing that it would just be another day of battling back and forth with him.

My stress level escalated when I tried to confide to my friend Jill about what was happening with David. She seemed detached and indifferent, yet strangely amused. This was new to me. I didn't understand why she reacted in that manner. It eventually became clear, but for now, Jill's close, happy, and positive friendship with me progressively started chipping away and would turn into a helter-skelter nightmare.

Weeks passed. My frustration grew. I left work each night feeling miserable. I worked part-time at a donut shop in the evenings. My steady customers and co-workers noticed and asked me why I was unhappy. I explained to them what was going on with David and how I was thinking about quitting my job. They all listened sympathetically. Some tried to give me advice. Several conjectured with a wink that David was giving me a hard time because he had a crush on me. Absurd! Then they all started making bets amongst themselves: one day David and I would be together as boyfriend and girlfriend. Absolutely ludicrous!

The busy season for our department entailed much more work than usual with year-end bonuses, direct deposits, forms such as W-2s, W-4s, and so on. It meant long days and nights and much turmoil in the office. Ironically during the busy period my relationship with David changed for the better. It seemed along the way we made a truce. He recognized what a hard worker I was, and my ability to multi-task went far beyond his expectations. I thanked God for that small miracle; otherwise, my extended hours with him would have been absolutely unbearable.

Strangely, the easier it was with David, the more difficult it was with Jill. She no longer asked me to go out for lunch or

dinner. When I asked her why she couldn't go, she used the
excuse that she was too busy. I learned from coworkers that
she was having lunch with David and now her weekends were
being spent showing David around New York City. She never
told me any of this; she just quietly dropped me as a friend. I
didn't understand why she was being secretive. I didn't care if
she went out with David. It troubled me that Jill was putting
a wedge in our friendship. Most importantly I didn't comprehend why she felt she had to lie to me. I decided I should ask
her to make time to talk with me, and this time I wouldn't take
no for an answer. I explained that I thought our friendship
had changed and we should discuss it. She agreed.

We decided to go to The Bridge, a rustic-looking bar and
grill where all the Wall Street Yuppies went for lunch or for
drinks after work. The food was good and it was a great place
to hang out and play darts. I sat across from Jill wondering
why on earth she couldn't look me in the eye. The place was
busy and very loud and perhaps she was distracted. I began
by asking her first if everything was all right with her. Was
she feeling well? Was anything troubling her? She responded
by saying she was feeling fine but there was something she
needed to tell me. Instantly I became alarmed. I wasn't sure
what she was going to say. Had I done something wrong?
She had been my friend and mentor. I was so nervous. She
proceeded by saying she had strong feelings towards David
and was possibly falling in love with him. I wondered what
this revelation had to do with me and with our friendship. She
continued that she hoped that I didn't share the same feelings
for David, and if I did, I needed to back off.

"Back off?" I thought to myself, "How dare she?" I felt
accused, shocked, and perplexed by what she was saying. Me?

Have romantic feelings toward David? Jill was definitely losing it! Trying to calm her down I reassured her that David was the furthest thing from my mind. Lately I had been neutral about David after working so hard to overcome my frustration with him. I told her I was surprised to learn that she had developed such strong feelings towards David because he was much younger than she was, and she hardly knew him. Jill misinterpreted my stunned reaction as if I was guilty of something. She voiced her own suspicions that David and I were dating. I insisted it wasn't true; an office rumor was circulating that David was interested in me. I even laughed a little and added, if David was interested in dating me, he had a funny way of showing it! Besides, the feelings weren't mutual. I reminded her I was still dating my boyfriend.

She demanded to know how my relationship with David had changed from conflicted to amicable. I explained that it was gradual. David and I were just trying harder to get along so it would be more tolerable for us to work with one another during the busy season. She didn't believe me. She continued to batter me with false accusations. I became upset and totally exhausted from trying to defend myself; I shut down and withdrew, as it had become extremely difficult to continue with the conversation. Nothing I could do or say could restore the friendship. Once lunch was over and we walked out the door of the Bridge, our relationship would change forever.

Several weeks passed after my talk with Jill. We were still civil to one another but everyone in the office could tell there was tension between us. I tried not to think about it too much. It was stressful enough with the year-end work. My personal life with my boyfriend was cooling down. Painfully

I wondered if it was going to last, but I kept my head up high and tried my best to stay positive.

A few nights a week after work some of the girls from the office, Mary Ellen, Terry, and I would go Christmas shopping for the office grab-bag. I had developed a close relationship with them since they were just about my age. They expressed concern and felt terrible for how my friendship with Jill had changed, but they couldn't resist teasing me about David. They strongly believed he had a thing for me. I asked them both why they thought that. The answer was simple, "It's the way he looks at you." I made a mental note to start being aware of it. Was I blind? Why didn't I notice it? It distressed me that this was going on and I didn't even have a clue. I was so caught up in the other things in my life that it never occurred to me that David and I could be an item.

I decided to have a serious talk with my best friend Stacie. Stacie and I had first met months before on the train while on our way to work. Each day I would stop at the little corner shop by the train station to get a tea and a newspaper. Stacie and I would see each other every morning but we never said anything more than a brief "Good Morning." Since I'm not a morning person the train and ferry ride into Manhattan was "my time." I never engaged in conversation; I would just enjoy my hot cup of tea and read the newspaper or a good book. That routine would be short-lived. One fine day Stacie sat next to me on the train and approached me by asking me where I worked. I gave her a sidelong look and answered, "Thomson McKinnon." I went back to my book.

She beamed this beautiful smile and said, "So do I!" She then asked, "Do you work in the Waffle Building?" Our office building was called the Waffle Building because it had little squares as windows which provided a waffle effect.

I replied, "Yes I do. I work in the Payroll Department."

She offered, "I work in Margins. Maybe one day we could go to lunch." Needless to say, we became best friends. After twenty-eight years Stacie and I are still best friends despite the miles between us. When we get together she still knows to give me my quiet time in the mornings.

One night on our way home from work I asked Stacie if she wanted to go for a ride back into the city. I needed to talk to her. We often drove into the city in the evenings just to unwind and go uptown to people-watch and admire the buildings. New York City is absolutely beautiful in the evenings especially during the Christmas season. She said yes. I said, "I'll pick you up in an hour." I went home to change into my sweats and sneakers. I hardly wore them anymore since I had become more proficient walking in my crazy-looking high heels. As I drove to Stacie's I remembered how she told me that when she first saw me on the train she thought I was a stuck-up fashion maven. She said I looked unapproachable dressed-to-the-nines each morning, totally reserved and mysterious. Stacie admitted that if she hadn't been so sassy she would have never talked to me. I laughed. I wasn't stuck-up. It was just that I wasn't a morning person, and I loved to wear the latest trends.

The night was bitterly cold. I expected Stacie to wear her sweats. Instead, she got into the car wearing flannel pajamas and big fluffy slippers. That was Stacie!

I remarked, "We're definitely not getting out of the car with you wearing that get-up!"

She laughed and handed me a mug of hot chocolate with extra marshmallows, declaring, "Now we are ready to go!"

Stacie was great like that. She knew that the hot chocolate and the spontaneity would make me smile. We were off to find Trump Tower. It had just been built and we were curious about it since it received so much attention. I'd read in Cosmopolitan magazine that Donald Trump was a multimillionaire, the Bachelor of the Month. We parked in front of the building. We were both in awe. The building was absolutely beautiful. It sparkled in bronze, gold, and marble. We wondered what type of people would come in and out of that building. We sat there people-watching. After a few minutes Stacie asked me what had been troubling me lately. I proceeded to tell her about all the rumors in the office and recounted my discussion with Jill. Stacie smiled with that beautiful smile of hers and began to laugh.

"Why are you laughing?" I asked.

"How can they think you like David?" she exclaimed. "They're all crazy! He isn't your type; his hair isn't long enough! He doesn't look like a rock star; he is a clean-cut executive!" I started to laugh with her. She was right. Why should I get so uptight about a rumor? I should stop wasting my tears and energy on the whole situation.

She also challenged me, "And why are you so torn up about your friendship with Jill? Forget about her; she isn't worth it. Besides, you have me now!"

I acknowledged, "Thank God." I turned to her, stronger now, and declared, "Stacie, I'm going to get out of the car. I want to go up to the building and peek through the glass doors. Maybe I'll get a glimpse of Donald Trump. Are you coming? I dare you to get out in your pajamas!"

Laughing, she said, "No, but go ahead. I'll stand here by the car." Approaching the building I looked back, and there was

Stacie standing by the car in her pajamas and fluffy slippers as beautiful, well-dressed women in fur coats walked by.

By the first week of December my boyfriend and I had broken up. Although I had seen this coming I was extremely upset and very hurt. It had been difficult not being able to show any emotions at work and keep myself together during the day. I was working late hours at night and still at the donut shop on the weekends. I was totally exhausted and emotionally drained.

One evening everyone but me had gone home from the workplace. I was waiting in my office for a cab to pick me up. I had some time so I picked up the phone and called my big-brother friend, Johnny. He had been consoling me through the break-up with my boyfriend, trying to give me a guy's perspective on things. He always had a way of making me feel better. But on this particular night I was inconsolable. When the phone call ended, I leaned on the edge of my desk with my back towards the front door of the office. Covering my face with my hands, I closed my eyes and quietly wept. Alone, I poured out my heart and soul unleashing the pain. I released all the stress that I'd held inside for weeks. Through my sobs I never heard David approach. With my head down I let the tears fall. As I wiped my tears and opened my eyes I was surprised to see his shoes. David was standing in front of me. I slowly looked upward until my gaze reached his beautiful blue eyes. Our eyes locked. He looked at me intensely, insistently, wiping a tear from my cheek. He asked, "Why are you crying? What could possibly be so wrong?"

I couldn't find my voice to even answer him. I could feel my heart pounding in my chest. I was astonished to see him standing there. I suddenly felt very vulnerable and self-conscious. I frantically looked away from him. I looked down at the floor. I didn't know what to do. In my wildest dreams I never anticipated nor could I predict his next move. He stepped forward and closed the distance between us. He lifted my chin up very slowly, looking deeply into my eyes, and without a word spoken between us he gently touched my lips with his. It was a kiss that was so sweet and so tender that I felt my body relax, accepting the comfort of his kiss. Just as quickly, alarms went off in my head. My brain was screaming, "No! No! No! This can't be happening! Why is my body responding? We are coworkers." I retreated, looking away. My heart thumped and I felt like I was going to pass out…My rapid breathing told me this was wrong. Confusion and amazement overwhelmed me. Dazed and shaken to the core, I gathered my things, escaping to the taxi waiting outside for me.

Follow the way of love...

—1 CORINTHIANS 14:1

CHAPTER TWO

David had kissed me. I couldn't believe he had actually done it. It took my stunned brain a second to absorb that fact. I sat in the back seat of the cab with my heart still pounding and my pulse racing. I leaned my head against the head rest and closed my eyes reliving the kiss. It was strange; I felt exhilarated and sick to my stomach at the same time.

This was going to complicate our relationship even further. Did he understand the implications? Didn't he know that it went against work ethics? What about Jill? What would happen if she found out? How was I going to face him the next day? All these unanswered questions made my head hurt. I needed to get home, crawl into bed, and take some quiet time to sort things out. In the morning I would talk to Stacie; she would give me some advice.

With much trepidation I went to work the next day. Boarding the train Stacie took one look at me and knew something was wrong. "Are you OK? You look tired."

I answered, "I didn't sleep well last night." Then I told her what had happened the night before. Stacie looked at me incredulously and began to laugh. In my opinion there was nothing funny about it... I wanted to "kill" her. "No, Stacie, this is serious. In less than an hour I will be walking through that office door." Needless to say Stacie found my story thrilling and exciting. She encouraged me to keep an open mind and explore my options.

Anticipating the Christmas party that afternoon, I had convinced myself that perhaps there would be a lot of hustle and bustle and I wouldn't come in contact with David. No such luck. As I entered the office I saw him helping an employee of another department. I glanced at him quickly, hoping he wouldn't notice me. At that same moment he looked up and our eyes met and locked. Smiling, he said, "Good Morning."

I smiled back and responded, "Good Morning." I felt dizzy; I thought I was going to faint. I had butterflies in my stomach and my heart began thumping as I walked to my desk. I remember thinking: Wow, he really does have such pretty eyes and a nice smile. Why was I suddenly noticing all these things about him?

I managed to keep myself busy all morning. The holiday lunch was being catered, and gifts would be found in the grab-bag. We had to guess which gift belonged to us. There were no names on the name tags; the person giving the gift had to write something describing that person.

One box said, "She has rings on her fingers and bells on her toes, she types music wherever she goes." I had rings on every finger except my thumbs. I found it very fashionable and it became part of my persona. It made me unique and different. When someone had to refer to me they would say, "The girl with all the rings on her fingers."

David had given each member of the staff a gift with a Christmas card. Jill had made a big deal letting everyone know she had helped him choose the gifts and helped him wrap them. Each of us received a coffee mug with a word on one side and the definition on the other side. David enjoyed stuff like that. For example, his daily calendar was "The Word of the Day."

Since a few people in the office had opened their gift I wasn't too eager to unwrap mine. Later in the day, Mary Ellen and Terry approached my desk and noticed that I hadn't opened mine yet. They coaxed me, "Open it! Open it!" They were curious to see what word was on my mug. I told them that I was sure that the mugs were random, and the word wasn't chosen individually. They insisted I open it. Just to satisfy them I did so. When I pulled the mug out of the box, our jaws fell open. The word on my mug was LOVE!! I sat there stunned and wide-eyed. Mary Ellen and Terry started giggling. I wanted to crawl under my desk and hide. They started teasing me by saying, "Oh I'm sure the mugs were randomly given to us." And, "Imagine if Joe in the office would have received that one." I wanted to "strangle" them both. When they walked away from my desk, I immediately put it in my drawer so no one else could see it, in particular Jill.

With my hands trembling, I opened up my Christmas card from David. I figured since I couldn't keep the mug on my desk I would display his card instead. Once again I sat there in shock. I couldn't believe my eyes. I read it twice, three times, to make sure I wasn't hallucinating. The card read on top, "Dear Michelle," and on the bottom it said "If you ever decide what you want out of life, you know where to find me." Feeling flustered I took the card and walked over to Mary Ellen's cubicle. I placed the card on her desk and said, "Read this."

She opened it up and read it. She looked up at me with a big grin on her face and said, "I told you he had a thing for you. What are you going to do about it?"

I answered quietly, "I don't know. I'm not sure how I feel about him. Or the situation." I slowly walked back to my desk, hoping the day would end quickly. Inwardly I thought, wait until I show Stacie the card—she's going to get a big charge out of it. Believe me, she did. Once again she encouraged me to go out with him and get to know him out of the work setting.

The holidays passed. The next few months were uneventful. The office slowed down considerably. My days working with David improved. We were finally getting along. The tension between us seemed to dissipate and was replaced by a delightful sense of discovery. Some days we would laugh and joke privately. The battling between us changed into a friendly bantering. When he reviewed my work it wasn't with a critical eye, he gently made suggestions. Throughout the day I would find a little something on my desk. Certain mornings there would be a package of cookies or my favorite donut. There were days he would leave a candy bar, chips or a drink, and occasionally I would find the word-of-the-day up on my bulletin board—"rambunctious" for one. I started to realize I was looking forward to these small gestures.

I was more conscious of my appearance and if there was anything I could tweak, I did so, hoping he would notice. Oh, and he noticed. He was always complimenting me on how nice I looked. I wore my makeup a little differently, outlining my eyes with eyeliner to make them look like cat eyes. One day, David was dictating a letter to me. In mid-sentence he stopped. I looked up, catching his gaze. "What is wrong?"

He stared at me intently. "You have such beautiful brown eyes."

I smiled. Feeling a little nervous I challenged, "How about Jill? Don't you think she has pretty blue eyes?"

He shook his head. "No, yours are absolutely incredible." I blushed; my heart quickened. There was definitely something developing between us. Inwardly I was thinking how I would like to get to know him outside of the work environment.

That's exactly what I did. It was one of those nights that Stacie and I would take one of our famous rides to unwind. Our destination this time was New Jersey. I wanted to go to the Woodbridge Mall to buy a pair of boots at my favorite shoe store. On the way out of the mall Stacie and I grabbed a coffee and a hot cocoa for the ride home. I was driving on the New Jersey Turnpike unaware that I had driven past the exit that I needed to get to the outer bridge towards Staten Island. Stacie asked me, "Where are you going?"

"What do you mean? I'm heading home."

She laughed, "Really? That's funny; we just drove by all of the exits to Staten Island."

When I approached the next exit, I looked to see what number it was and realized that she was right. With a sly smile on my face I glanced at her and said, "I guess I'm heading north to David's." David lived in Cliffside Park. I wasn't sure what I was going to do or what to expect once I got there. We pulled up in front of his place and parked. We sat there for a few minutes like a couple of teenagers just staring at the two-story building wondering which apartment he lived in. The upper apartment had the TV and lights on.

Stacie looked at me. "OK, so now what? Do you think he lives in the upstairs apartment?"

I shrugged my shoulders. "I'm not sure. I guess we will have to sit here for a little while and see if we see him through the window."

Stacie snorted. "Sit here? Tell me we just didn't drive all this way to sit here. I double dog dare you to ring his doorbell." I gave her my most menacing look.

"I can't believe you just dared me to do that. You know I never shy away from a dare."

She laughed and sing-songed, "I'm waiting…we don't have all night."

As I got out of the car I looked back at her. "Get out of the car—you are coming with me. And thank God you are not wearing pajamas and fluffy slippers." We approached the building. We guessed he lived on the second floor. My hands were clammy. The sound of my pounding heart roared in my ears. I looked at Stacie in a panic and whispered, "I can't do this"

Smirking, she challenged me, "Why? Are you scared? Well, I'm not." She then very eloquently pointed her finger at the doorbell and rang it. I could have screamed.

David's voice came over the intercom, "Who is it?" I hesitated a moment. Stacie nudged me with her elbow.

Timidly I offered, "It's Michelle."

David responded immediately, "Come up." My entire body started to tremble. I didn't even know if I could walk up the stairs. I froze in place.

Stacie grabbed my arm and pulled me inside the building. I hissed at her, "Stop it! I need to take a deep breath and compose myself. I feel like I'm going to have a heart attack!" She stood there laughing, waiting patiently. We proceeded up the stairs. As we rounded the landing, I looked up and there he was, waiting for us in the doorway with a big smile. At that moment we both felt the connection between us and knew our relationship was going to change.

Dating David proved to be extremely challenging as well as exciting. Our relationship had to be kept a secret because it was against work ethics and of course we had to keep it from Jill. Our first real date was absolutely incredible. I remember him asking me out to dinner after work one night. We walked up Broadway to a restaurant called Winston's. I was flattered and surprised he was taking me there. It was a very expensive place to eat. The bigger surprise came when we were escorted to the upper level of the restaurant where no one else was seated. This level overlooked the first floor. A piano man played soft music. It was absolutely romantic. I noticed after a little while that the maitre d' purposely wasn't seating anyone where we were. I brought it to David's attention. He smiled and nodded, "I know, I requested him to do that if he could."

I smiled back, "How did you manage that?"

Still grinning at me he said, "It's not important how I did it. I told him it was a very special night." The evening was incredible. Dinner was great and so was David's company. I couldn't have asked for anything more perfect. One last surprise, as we were relaxing and enjoying our drinks, the piano man started to play a song. I found myself humming to it. I suddenly realized it was one of my favorite classical songs. A soft smile appeared on my face. David tilted his head. "Why are you smiling?"

Shyly I responded, "I love this song. It's the theme song of Romeo and Juliet, one of my favorites. I know you think all-I-listen-to is heavy metal, but there are many things about me you don't know."

He laughed aloud. "I know it's your favorite. I asked him to play it for you. I overheard you tell Mary Ellen. Since I don't know you all that well, I would love to get to know you better and make it official. Will you go out with me?" At that moment my heart was filled with happiness. I looked deeply into his eyes and responded.

"Yes, I would love to."

David and I created a state of bliss. Every moment we had

outside of work we spent together. Since he was new to the area we did a lot of things in the city. I would meet him on the weekends, and we would go to the Village, better known today as Tribeca. We went to Times Square, Central Park, etc. We took pleasure in simple activities, just walking, window shopping, eating at little hole-in-the-wall restaurants, or simply just sitting on a park bench, eyes closed, holding hands with the sun hitting our faces. On other occasions I would go to David's house in New Jersey. We would go motorcycle riding, cook dinner together, or occasionally spend a quiet night watching TV if his roommates weren't home.

We were slowly growing together as a couple. Although our weekends were awesome, working together became increasingly difficult because we had to watch every move we made. It was challenging sometimes separating our personal life from our professional one. We managed to keep it from the others for several months. Jill's suspicions mounted. David was no longer hanging out with her on the weekends. When she called me to go out for lunch or on the weekends, I made myself unavailable. One day, she noticed that David and I had matching portable music players. She found that extremely unusual. She started to put the pieces of the puzzle together. As that was happening, her attitude changed drastically. She became extremely angry and very wicked, exuding nothing but ugliness.

Hatred stirs up dissension,
but love covers over all wrongs...

—Proverbs 10:12

Chapter Three

Jill's tormenting and evilness toward me had now begun. Her spitefulness came out subtly, almost imperceptibly, and increased over time. At first I didn't even notice. Personal things of mine started to disappear from my desk. I just thought the cleaning personnel were taking them. With taunting glances at me she would leave Hershey's Kisses on David's desk, or little notes asking David out to lunch.

On a professional level he had to accept her invitations. Occasionally I would run into them at the restaurant with Jill hanging all over him as David sat there straight as a board. One afternoon my friends and I were at the Bridge having lunch and playing darts. Some sort of commotion came from the stairway. I turned my head to see what was going on. Jill was drunk or acting drunk, pretending to lose her footing so she could fall and hold onto David. My eyes locked with his and he saw my anger and disgust. I wondered how much more of this I would tolerate.

Later I spoke privately with him. I asked him to please explain to me why every time I saw them at lunch, Jill was all over him. He reassured me he wanted nothing to do with her romantically. He had grown suspicious himself. It was just for my benefit she was pulling her little scenes. He further explained she was somehow getting information on where I was having lunch and she made sure that was where they would go. He suggested to me the next time she wanted to go to lunch he would choose the place. He did this several times, diverting her plans. When Jill realized what David was doing she became even more incensed, and her lashing out at me became worse. Since she was in charge of the computer-programming department she would erase all of the work that I inputted. Weeks of work would just disappear from my computer screen.

Paydays were the busiest days of the month. Phones would ring off the hook and employees would come to the department with questions about their paychecks. Since I was the secretary I was in charge of the phones in addition to my other responsibilities on payday. I always made sure to arrive a little earlier so I would be prepared. One payday I sat there enjoying a cup of tea, reading the letters that needed to be typed, when the phones started to ring. As usual I answered my phone by saying "Good morning, Thomson McKinnon, Payroll Department."

The person on the other end said hello. I responded, "Hello, how can I help you?" The person kept saying "Hello? Hello? Hello? Is anyone there?" I kept talking into the phone. The person couldn't hear me and hung up. Another call came in, and the same thing happened again. It occurred several times. Finally I ran to another desk when the phone rang to see if their phone was working and it was. I called maintenance for repairs. Meanwhile I spent most of the day running from desk to desk to answer the phone. I was exhausted. When Maintenance finally came to look at the phone, I was informed that there was nothing wrong with the wiring and when he screwed off the mouthpiece to check the inner part, he discovered the voice transmitter was missing. Someone had intentionally removed it from the phone. I was stunned. Who would do that? I looked around the office at my co-workers, and it was like a light-bulb came on in my head. Only one person: Jill. It then dawned on me that Jill took my stuff from my desk. Jill had deleted my work from the computer. (It wasn't a computer glitch or because I didn't know how to save my work.) At that moment I was personally offended and felt sick to my stomach. I wondered who I could tell. I couldn't trust anyone in the office. An unknown colleague was telling her where I was going to lunch. I wasn't sure I could go to David. I didn't want him to think I was just pointing fingers at Jill. Although I was convinced she was deliberately trying to piss me off hoping I would get tired of her nonsense and break off with David, I decided to keep my thoughts to myself. I simply made a mental note to be more aware of her and my surroundings.

The following weeks I was hyper-vigilant, constantly on edge, and wary throughout the workday. I withdrew slightly from David. As time went on, the fact that I couldn't share my suspicions with him made me withdraw from him further. David did not understand. He saw the change in me and in our relationship. He constantly asked me if there was "something going on" or whether he had "done something wrong." I avoided his questions and never mentioned Jill.

One day I saw through his office window Jill alone with David in a meeting behind closed doors. I became absolutely infuriated and I was taken aback by the strength of my emotion. At that moment I realized I was extremely insecure about my relationship with David and I was about to lose control. Since I could no longer function or think straight I had to make a decision on what to do. I contemplated taking a medical leave of absence from work.

My sister invited me to Italy to visit her and my Italian friends. It would give me a break and allow me to mend both body and soul. Also, I would be able to figure out how I really felt about David and what to do with our relationship. I mulled over the idea for a little while not being able to make a definitive decision until…I experienced the final straw.

One morning I wore a suit, a black linen long pencil skirt with a white matching linen jacket. It was one of my favorite outfits, and very expensive. I proceeded to my desk, glancing over into David's office. He looked up from his work, and said with a smile, "Good morning. You look nice."

I smiled back, "Good morning. And thank you." I pulled out my chair and sat down. As I rolled the chair closer to my desk, I noticed a wet feeling penetrating through my skirt. I stood up and looked at the black nylon chair. I didn't see anything. I felt with my hand to see if it was wet with water. It was wet, but not with water. Someone had poured black ink on it. My linen skirt was ruined. I stormed next door to Jill's office. I went in and slammed the door shut. I glared at her, pointing my finger, and said, "I'm done with your crap! I know what you have been doing, and you better back off. And if you don't I will tell your precious David what a sick woman you are and he will never look at you the same way again."

She glared back at me with such hatred in her eyes. It was the first time I realized that she didn't have pretty blue eyes at all; they were a cold blue-grey and filled with hate. She pointed her claw-like nail at me and responded, "David is going to be done with you if you say anything to him. He is going to think you are nothing but an insecure, immature, jealous girlfriend. And when he is done using you he will put you on a shelf like a pretty little box to sit there to collect dust and rot. Then he will be with me."

I couldn't believe what I was hearing. I stood my ground and spat back, "You are twisted and you need help. There is no room in David's life for you. He is in love with me." I stormed out, slamming the door behind me. I went to the ladies room to look at my skirt. It was definitely ruined. I trembled with rage. The look on Jill's face had really scared me. I wondered what else she was capable of. At that moment I believed if she could find a way to further torment me, she would. I headed back and walked straight into my manager Len's office. I not only asked for the day off I also asked for a leave of absence. I did not bring up Jill. I would be gone at least a month.

It was official; I was leaving for Italy. It broke my heart to tell David but I decided he had to know now what was going on with Jill. I went into David's office, shut the door, and said to him "Are you going to be home tonight? I need to talk to you. It's really important." His expression was sad and perplexed. He could tell from the look on my face it wasn't going to be good. He answered, "Yes, why don't you come over for dinner? I'll cook for you." I explained I was going home because my skirt got ruined and I would see him later.

When I approached David's place I started to get nervous. I was hoping he would believe all I had to say. Dinner was great. His roommates weren't home, so it was nice and quiet, a perfect setting for a difficult conversation. I recounted the whole sequence of events with each and every suspicion, including what happened to me that morning and my talk with Jill. He was astounded. He expressed how hurt he was I didn't come to him earlier and that I made the decision without him to take a leave of absence. But on the other hand he was relieved because he wasn't sure what Jill would do next. Hopefully, my time away would ease the tension. He apologized for everything I had gone through. He felt responsible and blamed himself for all that had happened to me. We promised to keep in touch while I was gone. Saying goodbye wasn't easy. My eyes filled with unshed tears. We hugged each other tight and kept repeating how much we would miss one another. When he finally let go he took my face in his hands and kissed me goodbye. Unlike the first kiss which promised a new beginning, this kiss assured me he would be waiting for me when I came home. I sat in my car at the end of his street unleashing my tears, praying I had made the right decision.

And now these three remain: faith, hope, and love.
But the greatest of these is love...

— 1 Corinthians 13:13

Chapter Four

We were good on our promises. David and I spoke on the phone a few times while I was in Italy. He informed me that his relationship with Jill was much different, describing it as cool and professional.

My trip to Italy was incredibly refreshing. I spent time with friends with whom I'd become acquainted in years past when visiting my sister, and found myself again. I revisited the region of Tuscany and the Italian Riviera. It was exactly what I needed.

The Italian men were great for my ego. They were just as charming and lovable as their country. Although I was having the time of my life I sorely missed David. Being away from him I didn't know what was left of the relationship. If I had to be honest with myself I was never really sure where I stood with him; I was feeling so apprehensive about us. During my time away I had come to a decision. If he still wanted to date and was serious about me, I would consider changing jobs. That way we could date openly and have a normal relationship. Meanwhile, in the back of my mind I also had romantic thoughts of staying in Italy, finding a sexy Italian man, and living in the beautiful city of Florence. That city had enchanted and captured my heart, but it would remain a dream for the time being.

As my time in Italy came to an end, I felt the difficulty of leaving my sister and my Italian friends. I reassured myself I wouldn't wait so long to return. My travels in the past had also taken me to France, Monaco, and Monte Carlo but no other place was as beautiful as Italy. I knew of cities I still wanted to see—Rome being one of them, especially since I had not had the time to see it on this trip. I promised myself I would be back soon.

The weekend prior to returning to work I visited David at his place. It was great to see him. We had really missed one another and had much to talk about. He wanted to know all about my trip. I described in detail the beautiful cities I visited. I discussed with him my plans to look for a new job. I further explained it was extremely important that I know how he felt about me before I made such a drastic decision. He made it very clear he didn't want our relationship to end and yet he wasn't sure how we could continue with Jill always interfering. He felt bad I would have to change jobs in order for us to be together. There was no other choice; he was fairly new in his position so it wouldn't be advantageous for him to leave. The decision was final. I would actively start sending out my résumé. I was excited. It was time for me to explore my options and spread my wings.

Life moved very quickly during the next few months. David and I became closer with each passing day. We were always together and busy on the weekends. We took trips to upstate New York visiting where he once lived and had gone to college. He introduced me to his circle of friends. David slowly opened himself to me allowing me to be part of his life.

The big surprise came when he was invited to a wedding. He asked me if I would like to go with him. Since it was where his dad lived he would love for me to meet him. That invitation meant so much to me. His desire for me to meet his dad confirmed how he really cared about me. I was beginning to think I had made the right decision. Life seemed to be moving in the right direction.

My job search was extremely tedious. I went on interviews during my lunch hour or before work. There were two interesting positions; one was at Goldman Sachs and the other was at Solomon Brothers. The job at Solomon Brothers appealed to me. I would be the administrative assistant to the vice president of the department as well as for ten other men. Some of their offices were located in the same building I was currently working in. They also had offices at the World Trade Center and at 55 Water Street. When I received a phone call from the Human Resources Department of Solomon Brothers asking me to come for a second interview I was thrilled. After the interview I had a good feeling about it. Later that week they offered me the position and I accepted happily, knowing I would be free to date David openly. I couldn't wait to share the good news with David and my friend Stacie.

While I was away in Italy, Stacie had accepted a new position at a different company. She had met a guy and was dating him pretty seriously. She had met new friends from work and was hanging out with a different crowd. We were each doing our own thing. We still remained extremely close but at the same time we were moving on. I hoped for both of us that it was for the best.

It was in the month of May when I walked into my

manager's office to let him know I was leaving. It was going to be a very difficult conversation. Len had been good to me. He was a laid-back kind of a guy, never demanding too much from me, and always respectful and courteous. I enjoyed working with him. I hated to do this to him. I knocked on his door. He asked me to come in. I straightened my shoulders and proceeded inside. He looked up from his work and said "Hi, what's up?" I smiled.

I asked, "Are you busy? I would like to talk to you if you have some time." He gestured for me to have a seat. I sat down. I was trembling. We talked about work for a few minutes. Finally I plunged right into what I was there for. I informed him regretfully I was leaving and taking a job with another company.

Len frowned at me and said, "I didn't realize you were unhappy here."

I wished I could have told him everything but at this point it was senseless. I responded with a somber expression. "I'm leaving for a better position and a higher salary." I felt relieved I had finally said it.

He leaned back and looked at me intently. "Do you mind me asking what kind of position, and what did they offer you as a salary?"

I was a little perplexed and uncertain why he was asking me such questions. I had butterflies in my stomach. I wanted this conversation to be over. I managed a little smile and answered, "Administrative Assistant. And they offered me an increase of ten thousand dollars."

Len grinned broadly and offered, "Well, I don't see why we can't change your job title and match the salary." It took my breath away. My eyes widened in astonishment. I certainly didn't expect this. How could he even match it? That would be a huge raise in pay. He explained further, "Michelle, you have been a valued employee. I really don't want to see you leave. I'm sure David will agree with me. And of course we will have to get a final approval from Clark."

Surprised and touched, I couldn't utter a word. My eyes filled with tears. I had to say something quick. I stammered, "Len, thank you so much for your kind words and generous offer but I can't stay. It's time for me to apply my skills that I have learned here and grow with another company."

He seemed extremely disappointed. He nodded his head. "I understand. You will be sorely missed. If you change your mind please let me know."

I stood up and proceeded to my desk. I could feel the relief spread throughout my entire body. I was another step closer to a new life and freedom with David. It wasn't long until Jill got wind of the news. She pranced around like a peacock. It seemed as if a fire was turned on inside of her. Since I had returned from Italy, Jill and I hardly said two words to one another unless it was work-related. Every time she had to see Len and David, she passed by my desk. She never acknowledged me; she just walked by with a smug look on her face. In her sick mind she probably thought she had won the battle. She might have won "something" but I'm the one who had won David's heart.

My two-week's notice passed very quickly. The office gave me a going away party. I was really sad. I had met a lot of wonderful people during my time at Thomson-McKinnon. Certain colleagues gave me a little gift of remembrance. Jill had the nerve to do the same. She came over to my desk at the end of the party and tried to hand me a box. I looked at her, never taking the gift from her hands. She had a smirk on her face and placed the box on my desk. "Just a little something I picked up for you when I was in Haiti." I stared at her with no emotion on my face and didn't say a word. When she walked away, over her shoulder she said, "I hope you like it," and giggled. I took the box and threw it right in the garbage. Whatever was in the box seemed to be just as evil as she was. Today I often wonder what was in it.

Life seemed to finally begin for David and me. We could see each other openly. I felt such freedom. Our relationship was strong and solid. All my insecurities about us seemed to disappear. It was the happiest I had ever been.

My first few weeks at Solomon Brothers were hectic. I had much to learn and many people to meet. My boss Lou was great, as were the other guys in the department. They all showed patience and the will to give me a helping hand. I enjoyed the hustle and bustle of Wall Street. David would call me every afternoon for lunch. I looked forward to his calls. I always had a lot to tell him.

Although I enjoyed being busy at my new job I felt a little run down from the transition. When I had switched jobs I hadn't been able to take any time for myself. I was glad and relieved when David and I planned to go away for a long weekend around Father's Day. We were going to visit David's brother and wife in Philadelphia. They were expecting their first child. I had crocheted a baby blanket for a gift hoping to impress them. It was my first time meeting them and I was really excited.

My mom expressed her displeasure about me being away on Father's Day. She had a sense of foreboding. She begged me to stay home and spend the day with my dad. I normally would never give Mom a hard time—being brought up in a strict Italian family you didn't disobey your parents—but going away with David and meeting his brother were very important to me.

I wish today I listened to Mom. Ultimately this trip changed the whole course of my life. If I only had a crystal ball I could have seen what the future held for me. It was Friday June 13th, a beautiful summer day. Skies were blue, temperature was perfect. The drive to Philadelphia was great. I felt so relaxed, not a care in the world. I was going to spend the weekend with the man I loved. Life couldn't be any better. We had plans to visit the King of Prussia Mall and some of the famous historic sites Philly had to offer. We arrived late morning at David's brother's house but nobody was home. Apparently they were working and wouldn't be home until later that day.

David and I decided to go for a bike ride. It was a picture perfect day. We went downtown for lunch and window-shopped, and then we decided to ride the bike trail that runs along the Schuylkill River and expressway. The day was turning out to be pretty incredible. There we were riding side-by-side, laughing, talking, and being carefree when suddenly it came to an abrupt halt. Everything went wrong. Two bikers were coming towards us. They couldn't get past us and we had to get out of their way. David and I simultaneously had the same thought—we both accelerated, trying to get ahead of one another and our bikes collided. As I flew through the air I saw: sidewalk, river, sidewalk, grass, curb, a highway, and then my head struck the curb of the expressway and everything went dark.

When I awoke I was in the hospital. Everything hurt especially my head. David sat nearby waiting for me to wake up. I looked at him questioning, "What happened?"

With a worried expression on his face he began with, "How

are you feeling?"

I started to cry. "I hurt all over and I feel sick to my stomach."

He came over to my bed and took my hand. "Michelle, you are very lucky to be alive." I didn't understand what he meant. He tried to explain how close to death I came. He said I landed so near the highway that I could have been crushed to death with no chance of surviving.

Shaken with what he just told me, I took a deep breath, closed my eyes, and thanked God for his protection. I spent the rest of the weekend in the hospital. I had received several stitches on the side of my head. I also bruised several ribs and tore up my left knee pretty bad. They informed me I had suffered a seizure after I struck my head. The drugs that they were giving me were making me feel confused and extremely nauseous. I was in a daze. I was dehydrated from all of the vomiting. I waited a day to call my Mom to let her know what happened.

I recall telling my mom there was a drug by the name of Dilantin that they were giving me for seizures. It was making me extremely sick. She told me, "Stop taking the medicine and have them give you something else." Mom was very worried and wanted to make the trip to Philadelphia. I assured her that I was fine and would be coming home on Monday.

Needless to say our weekend was ruined. David spent most of the time at the hospital. I encouraged him to spend time with his brother and wife. There was nothing he could do for me. He remained loyal and stayed by my side. He felt guilty and responsible for what had happened.

I was released on Monday. When I was discharged I was instructed to see a neurologist to have a complete workup to make sure of no bleeds or clots and to get the stitches removed. The three-hour car trip home was absolutely miserable. I still hurt all over. David tried to make the ride home as comfortable for me as he could. He had placed pillows and blankets on my seat. I apologized and expressed how I was very upset that our perfectly-planned weekend turned out to be a disaster. He squeezed my hand and reminded me that we were going to have another get-away next month to Lakewood to visit his friends.

I closed my eyes feeling utterly reassured. At that moment it seemed the worst was over.

It was only the beginning. Nothing could prepare me for what was coming next.

Do not let your hearts be troubled and do not be afraid.

— JOHN 14:27

CHAPTER FIVE

We all have a bicycle injury in our lifetime and it is usually no big deal. Mine, on the other hand, is still causing me pain and suffering twenty-eight years later.

When I returned home from Philadelphia my mom was extremely concerned and upset. I never heard the end of it. She continually reminded me how she'd told me not to go to Philadelphia with David and how my place should have been at home with my dad. Mom is an incredibly strong Italian woman. Her heart is filled with love and her spirit is filled with fire. She can be headstrong when she feels certain about something. I wouldn't change a single thing about her; I wouldn't want her any other way. I assured her I was going to be fine despite how I looked after the accident.

I made doctors' appointments to follow-up my head injury. I did not want to prolong this. I wanted to complete it before David and I went on another weekend getaway. I was upset; the doctors frightened me. Did I have a blood clot on my brain? My first appointment was with my general physician to have my stitches removed. Then I would have to see a specialist for an evaluation of my head injury. It frustrated me to take time off from work for medical appointments. I had just started with Solomon Brothers. Fortunately my new boss was very understanding.

My family doctor had always been good to me. I believed he would know the best treatment because he knew my medical history. Unfortunately my stitches weren't ready to come out. He told me I would have to wait another week, and as bad luck would have it, he would be on vacation. He referred me to one of his colleagues across town. He also recommended that I see a neurologist for an evaluation. This was a disappointment as I had hoped that one doctor could take care of it all. No such luck; this was turning into a nightmare.

I had so many exciting plans for the following weeks and suddenly they were complicated with medical appointments. My oldest sister Teresa and my three nieces were coming from Italy at the end of June. I was looking forward to that; it was going to be nice to have a house full of family. I also anticipated my youngest sister Paulette's graduation from high school.

When I went to see my doctor's colleague a week later to get my stitches removed I had to explain to him all over again what happened. To my surprise he informed me the removal of my stitches was long overdue. Could these doctors get it right? And there would be no need for me to see a specialist. He said he could prescribe something for the seizure. I was skeptical of his lack of thoroughness and what he told me. I took his prescription for phenobarbital and threw it in my purse never intending to get it filled.

I contacted a neurologist to schedule a work-up due to the head injury. The only time available was on the day of Paulette's graduation. What a bind. If I didn't take the appointment I wouldn't be able to get in until late July.

On graduation day my mom wanted very much to accompany me to the neurologist's to show her support but I couldn't allow her to give up her moment of glory watching Paulette go across the stage to receive her diploma. She had waited so long for that to happen. I insisted I would be okay and it was much more important for Mom to be there for Paulette. Mom wasn't happy about me going to the doctor alone. Once again, her mother's intuition was telling her: something was going to go wrong for Michelle. But she knew she couldn't split herself in two. Paulette looked sharp in her cap and gown. I was so proud of her. We were close as sisters. Growing up with her was always an adventure. On her day of graduation Paulette was disappointed I wouldn't be able to make it to the ceremony. She thanked me for being there for her every step of the way. I told her that's what big sisters do. I kissed her on the cheek and went off to my appointment.

I felt apprehensive. I'd never been to so many doctors in my life. I was always a healthy child. My only downfall was that I was a very picky eater. As a result of that Mom always made sure she prepared for me special foods because she didn't want me to get sick. My brothers and sisters were always teasing me. She would make me a steak for dinner and they would have to eat pasta. They would taunt me by saying "Mommy spoils you," or "You are Mommy's favorite." Mom would explain that if she didn't make something special for me to eat I would get sick. They would protest and start complaining that they were tired of eating pasta, and they wanted special dinners too! That made Mom extremely angry. She would take out her wooden spoon and whirl it around in the air and yell, "If I could afford to feed you all steaks, I would!" They all shut up very quickly. They didn't want to get smacked with the wooden spoon.

When I worked both jobs I no longer had the luxury of having Mom's incredible dinners. Actually, there was no time to eat. I went from a healthy size ten when I started working at Thomson McKinnon to a size five at the time of my bicycle accident. As a consequence of my bad eating habits and all the stress at work, not only did I develop an ulcer I also had a few fainting episodes due to having borderline anemia.

The doctor introduced himself. He sat behind his desk and looked over the paperwork I had just filled out. He seemed rather unconcerned and started to ask me questions about the bike injury. I answered to the best of my ability. We spoke about my health history. I explained to him that I was a pretty healthy girl and the only problem was that I occasionally suffered with fainting spells due to the anemia. I told him that they were so infrequent it wasn't an issue at all for me. He frowned. "When you fainted, were there any witnesses?"

I answered, "Yes. One time I was on the train on my way home from work and my girlfriend was with me as well as a hundred other people. Another time I was lying in the sun. I went inside to grab something to drink. When I reached the kitchen I fainted. My Mom was there for that one."

"Did your girlfriend or Mom say if you went into a convulsive state?"

"No, they didn't witness anything like that."

"Do you understand what I mean by being in a convulsive state?"

"Yes. Like when someone is having a seizure."

He nodded his head and looked at my paperwork once again. When he looked up he said, "Well it says here that you suffered a seizure when you had your bicycle accident."

I said, "Yes, I was told I had a seizure, but *after* I struck my head on the concrete curb."

He proceeded, "Are you sure you didn't have a seizure first, and that is what caused you to have the bike accident?"

I straightened. "Yes, I'm sure. Our bikes collided and that is what caused me to fall."

He sat there quietly for a few minutes. "Well, I think you have epilepsy, and you are suffering with grand mal seizures." I looked at him in disbelief. Was he crazy? I wasn't an epileptic. He had it all wrong. I asked him how he derived that diagnosis. He explained in his opinion that my fainting episodes were seizures and I was just not aware of it, and I probably had one while riding my bike and didn't know it, and that is what caused me to fall.

I sat up in my seat even straighter and said in a firm tone, "No! That is not what happened. I had a seizure after striking my head. And I am not an epileptic. I faint due to anemia." I began to cry. I couldn't believe it; this was totally absurd. I wanted out of his office quick. I asked him if he had intentions of running any tests to confirm his diagnosis. He said he would do an EEG and a CAT scan, and some blood work to see what my levels were after taking the medicine for a month.

He also wrote me a prescription for phenobarbital. I couldn't believe my eyes…the same medicine the other doctor prescribed me. I sat there trying to control my emotions. I asked him what kind of medicine he was giving me and what were the side effects of it. He explained that phenobarbital was given for seizures. It has been around for a long time. It is so safe it can be given to babies. Side effects weren't bad at all. They included receding gum line, and it would make me feel very sleepy and tired. He tried to reassure me by saying, "You probably only have to take it for one year, always assuming you don't have any more seizures. You also have to be careful when driving while being on the medicine since it does cause drowsiness."

I explained to him I had started a new job that was extremely fast-paced. I couldn't feel tired while working. He said, "No problem," I could take my dosage at bedtime instead of throughout the day. That way I would get a good night's sleep.

I stood up, unsteady on my feet. I was dazed and confused, and still upset by what he'd just told me. I gathered my things and walked towards the door. He stood by the doorway waiting. As I approached he said to me, "Try not to be upset. There are a million people out there with epilepsy and they live a perfectly normal life."

But I didn't have epilepsy. He just didn't get it. In my heart of hearts I knew I wasn't an epileptic. I went to my car, got in, sat there and cried, wondering how all of this could be happening to me. I needed someone to talk to. I wasn't sure where I could go. I looked at my watch to see what time it was. Mom was still at the graduation. I started my car and put on the radio and began to drive aimlessly. It was one of those times when I needed to take a ride to clear my head. It always calmed me when I did that, especially since I had bought my Firebird the year prior. I felt it was my personal space and no one could intrude.

I found myself driving to an exclusive part of Staten Island. Todt Hill was a very prestigious neighborhood. I loved looking at all of the spectacular mansions. I often wondered who lived there and what they did for a living to afford these gorgeous homes. There was a rumor a mob boss lived in the area. I was curious to know if it was true and which house he lived in. As I drove up and down the streets it dawned on me that my sister-in-law lived nearby. I headed in her direction. I could talk to her about my doctor's appointment.

Glenda and I were very close. She was like an older sister to Paulette and me. When my brother Nick started dating Glenda she would bring cookies and donuts to us from the donut shop where they worked. She would also play board games with us like Monopoly and the game of Life. We thought she was the greatest thing since Barbie. When Paulette was nine and I was thirteen, it didn't take much to impress us kids. Glenda had a heart of gold. She was always kind and giving to our entire family. When I arrived at her house she opened the front door and immediately knew something was wrong.

Glenda and Nick had two handsome little boys and she was pregnant with their third child. They had asked me to be the baby's godmother. I was very excited about that. It would be my first time. Nicholas and Michael ran towards me yelling, "Aunt Mi-Mi, Aunt Mi-Mi!" I scooped them up, kissing and tickling them. When I was done playing with them Glenda brought them into the other room to watch TV. When she came back she sat next to me asking, "What is wrong? You don't look good."

I began to cry and explained what happened at my doctor's appointment. She stared at me wide-eyed in disbelief. She agreed with me that the doctor had misdiagnosed me. In all the years I was growing up, Glenda had never witnessed me having a seizure. I kept repeating over and over, "I don't know what to do. I don't want to take any medicine. I have a bad feeling about it. My gut is telling me no. I'm not an epileptic."

She took my hand trying to comfort me. "Then don't. You know you are not an epileptic. Who cares what he says." She was right. I didn't have to take anything. I would go and get the prescription filled and just not take it; then no one would ever know. I went to the pharmacy to get it filled. (During that era in 1986, a leaflet about side-effects was not provided to the consumer.) A month's supply was going to cost only $2.99. Good; the medicine wasn't going to cost me a fortune since I had no intention of taking it.

I drove home to tell Mom about my appointment. I was eager to see Paulette and hear all about her graduation. (To my disappointment Paulette wasn't home. She had gone with her friends to celebrate her day.) Mom was in the kitchen preparing dinner. I sat at the table listening to Mom about the graduation. She finally turned around to look at me and to ask how my doctor appointment went. When she saw my face Mom became alarmed. "What's wrong? What happened? You have been crying." I couldn't contain my emotions any longer. I burst into tears. She quickly walked over to me. Holding me close to her she repeated, "What's wrong? Please tell me. Are you OK?" I felt as if I was five years old. I didn't want her to let go. At that moment I wished she could just kiss me on my forehead and everything would go away. I looked up at her. She was wiping my tears away with her apron. She said soothingly, "Tell me what happened." I motioned for her to sit down. I knew she wasn't going to take the news well.

I held her hands saying, "The doctor said I'm an epileptic."

She jumped out of her seat. "Is he crazy? What would make him say that?" I explained to her that he came to that conclusion because of my fainting spells. That enraged her. She started to pace around the kitchen—ranting and raving in both Italian and English. She repeated over and over how she should have come to the appointment with me. She would have told the doctor that as a young girl she fainted because of anemia. No doctor had ever told her she was an epileptic. I finally calmed her down, getting her to sit in the chair. I hated to see her so upset. She looked into my eyes, so similar to her beautiful brown eyes, and said, "I should have come with you. I could have told him about your poor eating habits and how thin you have become in the last few months."

I assured her I had told the doctor about my eating habits and how much stress I was under. I said it didn't seem to make any difference to him. I further explained he was going to run some tests and he gave me medicine for seizures. The good news was, if I took the pills I would only be on them for a year if I didn't have any seizures. I added, "And Mom, we both know that won't happen because I'm not an epileptic." I gave her a big hug and told her not to worry about me because I would be OK. I knew that she needed to look forward to Teresa's arrival over the weekend and be prepared for a house full of grandbabies.

The weekend came and I was on my way to the airport to pick up Teresa and the girls. I couldn't wait to see them all. My oldest niece Jessica was eight, Jennifer was two, and baby Janet was going to celebrate her first birthday in July. All three of them were absolutely resplendent with different shades of red hair. They inherited that from previous generations of both sides of the family. Growing up, Teresa would always say she didn't want any kids with red hair so I guess God has a sense of humor. Although Teresa was nine years older, we were extremely close. Mom would talk about when Teresa was a little girl she would ask Mom for a baby sister, and she wanted to name her Michelle. She would always whine how Nick had Sal to play with, and she wanted a little sister to play with too. I was eleven when Teresa got married and moved to Italy. I was heartbroken whenever her brief visits ended. Her departure was always bittersweet. The next two months were going to be great having Teresa and the kids around.

The ride home from the airport was full of laughter and a lot of conversation. The girls couldn't wait to see their "Nonna" (Grandma.) Teresa asked me how everything was going after the bike accident. I briefly told her about the doctor's diagnosis of epilepsy. She was surprised. I confided in her that I didn't start the medicine and I wasn't sure if I would at all. I was so indecisive about what to do. All I knew was that I had a really bad feeling about taking it and that I should go with my gut feeling.

As each day passed I was increasingly looking forward to going on my next trip with David. I prayed it would be better than the last one. With everything that was going on I needed to relax and kick back. I made sure to schedule my tests for the coming week. That way they would be out of the way and hopefully I would have my results before I left.

I discussed the medicine situation with a few close friends. I told them I had to make a decision real soon on whether or not I was going to take the pills. In a month's time I would have to go for the blood work and I felt pressured and extremely troubled inside. I was in a constant battle with myself. I didn't know what the right choice was. My friends all had their own opinion about it. The one remark that frightened me the most was having a seizure while driving, possibly getting into a car accident and hurting or killing myself or someone else.

The decision was finally made when Mom found my untouched pills in my bedroom. She asked me why I had not taken them. I told her that I had a bad feeling about it. Teresa was sitting with us and she joined the conversation by telling me about a friend of hers in Italy. The friend was epileptic. She was taking phenobarbital and lived a perfectly normal life. I relented. The battle was over. I decided at that moment I would start taking the medicine.

The first few days on the medicine were uneventful. Life seemed normal. I was angry with myself for making a big deal about it. I went for my medical tests, the EEG and CAT scan. I was eager to know what the results were. I had to wait several days for them. As the days progressed I began to see changes, for example, it was getting more and more difficult to wake up in the morning. Before taking the medicine I had always arisen quickly when my alarm went off. Now I couldn't even open my eyes and I continually hit the snooze button. Mom noticed this happening. A few mornings she had to wake me up, get me out of bed, and into the shower so I wouldn't be late for work.

My work performance began to suffer. I was so fatigued I didn't have the ability to concentrate. I frequently took small breaks to go to the nurse's station to take quick naps so I could recharge and regroup. I couldn't continue on this path. I was concerned about losing my job. I decided to call the doctor's office to talk to them about what was going on and to find out my results, hoping if they came back normal he would discontinue the medicine or lower the dose. No such luck.

Although the results came back perfectly normal he wanted me to continue with the medicine. I was told that what I was experiencing is normal. My body needed to adjust to the medicine. Once it did, the effects would subside. I did what I was told. For once in my life, I wish I didn't.

I was driving home late one night from David's. I really wanted to spend the night with him but Mom totally disapproved. To avoid any discussions or arguments I made sure to go home. On this particular night I should have gone against Mom's advice and stayed over, dealing with the consequences the next morning. As I was driving on the New Jersey Turnpike I felt myself becoming increasingly tired. I had made sure not to take my medicine that night knowing I had to drive home. I tried everything to keep alert. My eyelids became heavy. I opened my windows a few inches. I put my radio on loud and I turned the air conditioner on high. Nothing prevented me from falling asleep behind the wheel. I drifted off for a few seconds.

I could feel the car pulling me to the left. My brain was screaming, "Wake up! Wake up!" I instantly opened my eyes. In front of me all I could see was the wall dividing the turnpike. I frantically turned my steering wheel to the right. I bounced off the wall, spinning out of control. I wasn't thinking of any possible cars behind me. The car did a 360 degree turn. I went into a panic. I waited for a car to hit me. I thought I was going to die. Scared and confused I tried to focus on what direction my car was heading. It was facing correctly south. I looked in the rear view mirror to see if there were any cars coming. Miraculously there were none. I pulled off the highway onto the shoulder of the turnpike. The car didn't feel right. It seemed to be off-balance. I wasn't able to steer the car; it was pulling me in the opposite direction. A loud noise came from the front on the driver's side. I didn't want to get out of the car to see the damage. I leaned forward grabbing the steering wheel and began to cry. My heart was pounding, my body shaking uncontrollably. I asked myself over and over, why, why was this happening to me?

I heard a tap on the driver's side window. I looked over. A

state trooper was standing there asking me if I was all right. I rolled down the window. He could see that I was crying. I explained what happened. He asked me if I had been drinking. I answered no. It alarmed me. I thought he was going to ask me to do a sobriety test. Instead he said, "You are very lucky to be alive. I saw the whole thing happen. I was sitting at the shoulder of the exit ramp and I thought you were going to hit the wall head-on."

I began to cry even harder. I asked him how badly was the car damaged. He took a step back to look and said, "Not a scratch. Your tire is a little tore up and hubcap a little bent. You probably bent your rim too." I couldn't believe it. I had to get out of the car to see for myself. At that moment I thanked God for my life and for no damages to the car. I didn't know how I was going to explain it to Mom.

The next few days the phenobarbital took a major toll on me. I wondered how much longer the effects would last. I physically started to slow down even further. It was becoming more difficult to do everyday tasks at home and at work. My lunch hour was now being spent in the nurse's office getting an hour of sleep. The only thing that kept me going was the anticipation that in a few days I would be going away with David. I continually reminded myself I could chill out and get some much-needed rest.

Mom wouldn't have approved, but the night before leaving for Lakewood I spent the night at David's place. We were going to get an early start. When I woke up the following morning I didn't feel well. I was extremely sluggish. My throat was sore and I felt feverish. I couldn't believe it. I hoped I wasn't coming down with the flu. I made my way into the bathroom to shower. I looked into the mirror to examine my throat. When I saw my reflection I realized my face was swollen especially around the eyes. There seemed to be some discharge in them. I went to David for his opinion. When he saw me he remarked about my face and eyes, how I could barely open them. He asked me if I wanted to cancel the trip since I wasn't feeling well. I said, "No, I'm really looking forward to getting away."

The drive up to Lakewood was absolutely miserable for me as my condition became worse. My fever was very high. It was a warm summer day and I was freezing, lying down in the passenger seat. David had put jackets over me to try to keep me warm. My throat felt like it was on fire. I was having difficulty swallowing. I attempted to drink water and nearly choked.

We had planned to stop and visit the town where David went to college. He decided we would seek medical attention from the nurse on campus. I drifted in and out of sleep. The ride there seemed to take forever. David gently woke me up and announced we had arrived. I could barely get out of the car. My entire body hurt. My vision was extremely blurred. With David's help I made it to the office. Regretfully, they weren't allowed to treat me. I wasn't a student of the college and it went against their school policy. We both decided to drive the rest of the way to our friend's house and figure out what I should do from there. As I drifted off to sleep my last thought was tomorrow will bring new promises and everything will be much better.

When we arrived at our friends' Rick and Julie's house, my condition had not changed. Julie took one look at me and knew I wasn't well. She helped me into the house. Showing me to my room I sat on the bed and started to cry. I hurt all over. I was feeling terrible. Julie asked if I wanted to go to the hospital. I explained my symptoms to her expressing how I thought that I just had the flu and all I probably needed was some rest. She suggested I lay down. When I awoke, if I wasn't feeling any better, she recommended maybe going to the convenience clinic. I agreed. I woke up an hour later. I was soaking wet. The fever was really high. I needed medical attention.

Julie and I drove to the clinic. The place was filled with people. We signed in and waited. I began to moan. I was doubled over from excruciating pain. I could barely see out of my eyes. Julie put a few chairs together so I could lie down and be more comfortable. After waiting a long while I became impatient. I begged Julie to ask them to get me in quicker. There was nothing they could do. I had to wait my turn.

I became irate. It was so unlike me. I got up, went to the nurse's window, and banged on it. I began to make a scene. I became loud, telling the nurses I had been sitting out there for two hours, repeating (from nowhere) how I thought I was having an allergic reaction to a medicine and I needed to see a doctor right now. I further told them how they should allow the more critical patients to go before the less critical. To avoid any further embarrassment they brought me into the back. I waited in the room for the doctor to come in. I was lying on the table in a fetal position. I kept thinking something was seriously wrong. This couldn't just be the flu. Why had I blurted out that I was having an allergic reaction to a medicine? Where the heck did that come from? Was my body telling me something? I made a mental note to discuss it with the doctor.

I had dozed off when the doctor finally came in. He took my vital signs, my temperature, and swabbed the back of my throat. He diagnosed me with strep throat. I mentioned my thoughts of an allergic reaction or a drug interaction. He didn't think that was the case. He wanted to give me a shot of penicillin. Before doing so, he asked me if I was allergic to penicillin. I told him "My brother is allergic to it. I've never been on it before. I have taken ampicillin and amoxicillin." He informed me they were all in the same family and I would be OK with it. Before he left he told me I would feel much better tomorrow. Just get rest and a lot of fluids. I was relieved to hear that. I was glad my whole weekend wasn't going to be ruined once again.

We had plans to go to a show at the performing arts center that evening. It was obvious to everyone I wasn't going anywhere. They all decided not to go either. They weren't comfortable leaving me home alone as sick as I was. I felt so guilty knowing I was going to spoil everyone's evening. I insisted I would be okay. All I needed was a good night's rest. I convinced them by telling them it was only strep throat and by tomorrow I would feel better and would be able to enjoy the rest of the weekend with them.

Before leaving they made sure I had a cooler by my bedside filled with water and juice. David was reluctant to leave me. He begged me to let him stay. I wouldn't allow him to do that. They had paid a lot of money for the tickets. David wasn't happy with my decision. He kissed me on my forehead and said "Get some rest. I love you, and I will see you in a little while."

In my haze I responded "I love you too. When you get back you'll see I will be better." Everyone left that evening with misgivings.

At some point I woke up having to use the bathroom. I tried to focus on my surroundings. I wasn't sure where I was. I was burning up. My fever had spiked. I was delirious. I couldn't stand up straight. I got on my hands and knees to crawl to the bathroom. I was using my hands to find my way. When I found the toilet I could barely sit on it. I was swaying off of it. I held onto the sink in order to keep my balance. In the distance I heard the doorbell and a knock at the door. In that moment of my delirium it didn't register to make my way to answer it. I just sat there. I thought I was hearing things. Why would they be knocking? Didn't they have a key? I continued to sit there. I leaned my head against the sink. I still wasn't sure where I was.

Once again the doorbell rang and the knock at the door was frantic. Someone was calling my name. I got on my hands and knees crawling to where the noise was coming from. I followed the sounds. I could hardly see out of my eyes. I made my way down the hallway. I began to yell over and over, "I'm coming. Please help." I finally made it to the door. I was feeling for the handle to pull myself up to unlock it. They kept calling out my name "Michelle! Michelle! Are you OK?" In my haze I tried to listen to their voices. I didn't recognize them. It wasn't Julie, David or Rick. Who were they? How did they know my name? Before unlocking the door I asked them, "Who are you?"

The voice responded, "It's Janet and Rick, Rick's parents. Please open the door." I was so relieved to know someone was there to help me. I opened it and collapsed on the floor. I felt strong hands picking me up, helping me to the couch.

I asked them, "How did you know to come?" Janet explained she had spoken to Julie earlier and knew how sick I was. Julie had asked her to check on me. Being a retired nurse she said my symptoms raised red flags. She also expressed how unhappy she was that they went out leaving me alone. She took my temperature; it was extremely high. That would explain my delirium. She put cool compresses on my forehead to try to soothe me. She told me I needed to go to the hospital when they got back. After a while they came home. I heard in the distance Janet saying in a firm voice how unhappy and disappointed she was that they had left me home alone and how I needed to get to the hospital immediately. David helped me to the car. Julie came with us. On the drive to the hospital I began to hallucinate. I thought Julie was a nurse. I wasn't sure who David was. When we arrived they got me right into the emergency room. David stayed behind to fill out all of the paperwork. I was in and out of consciousness. Julie was constantly by my side. In a moment of lucidity I looked at my arms as I was lying on the gurney. I saw little red spots appearing on my left hand, quickly traveling up my arm. I turned to Julie in a panic and said, "Look Julie. Look at my arm. These red spots are traveling all over my body." Julie looked at my arm and became alarmed. She quickly left the room to get someone to look at them.

Once again I lost consciousness. The next time I awoke it was the next day. I was in a regular room. They had admitted me. I looked around trying to get my bearings. I felt sick. The pain was unbearable. I was supposed to be better, not in a hospital. I still didn't know what was wrong with me. A nurse assisted me to the bathroom. Walking seemed like such a chore. I went to the sink to wash my hands. I looked into the mirror. I screamed. It wasn't my reflection. I had large blisters all over my face. In disbelief I placed my finger on one of them. The blister popped. I screamed aloud, "Oh my God! What is happening to me?" At that very moment my Mom was walking into my room. She heard my screams. She ran towards the bathroom. I saw her as I was coming out. "Ma, look at my face! I look like a monster!" She reached out and held me, and reassured, "Don't worry. You are going to be OK."

I will not keep silent; I will speak out in the anguish of my spirit, I will complain in the bitterness of my soul.

—Job 7:11

Chapter Six

Mom and Dad's ordinary life was about to change forever. Their glorious Saturday morning on Staten Island had begun differently from mine. Mom was washing the dishes from breakfast when the phone rang. She hurriedly went to pick it up assuming I would be checking in. "Hello?"

At first she didn't recognize the man's voice. It was David. He was saying something about Michelle being in the hospital and needed Mom to come to Lakewood quickly. It was very serious. The hospital personnel were asking him all sorts of questions about our family medical history and he didn't know how to answer them. Mom went into panic mode. All she heard was, "Michelle is in the hospital and it is very serious." She became upset and responded angrily.

"David, why is Michelle in the hospital again? What happened this time?" In her agitated state she didn't even hear his response. She asked him for directions to the hospital and barely heard them. She slammed the phone down. With her mind whirling in a million directions she looked for Dad. They would have to leave immediately. Mom found him tending to the garden. She ran out into the back yard, tears streaming down her face, yelling his name

"Nello! Nello! Michelle is in the hospital! We have to go to her *adesso* (now)!"

The drive seemed endless. Mom and Dad weren't sure how to get there. Before they left, my brothers and sisters had tried to explain to them it was the same way they would go to visit a cousin in upstate New York, only a different exit. With each passing mile, so many unpleasant thoughts crossed Mom's mind. She was overwhelmed with worry. She prayed in her head for God to get them there quickly. As they approached the exit Mom's anxiety mounted. Uncertain which direction to turn off from the highway, they made a left, hoping it was correct. After driving a while they were to look for certain landmarks letting them know they were close; no landmarks appeared. Dad stopped at a gas station and asked for help. He learned they were headed in the wrong direction and had gone forty-five minutes out of the way. Mom slumped in her seat and started to cry. She felt frantic. It seemed as if they would never get there. She didn't know what my condition was or whether I was going to make it.

She told me later, "I was never so happy to see the hospital in front of me." She went inside, going straight up to my floor. She asked the nurses at the desk which room was mine. They pointed right in front of their station. At the very same moment she heard a scream coming from the room. She recognized it to be mine; she ran in. There before her eyes, I was being assisted by a nurse. Mom was in disbelief. Her heart tore in two. My entire face was distorted by large blisters. I saw her and cried out, "Ma, look at my face. I look like a monster!" Mom reached out and embraced me, reassuring me that I was going to be OK. She helped the nurse put me back into bed. She told the nurse she wanted to speak to the doctor. The nurse informed her he was going to make his rounds about seven o'clock. She looked at her watch. It was five o'clock.

My mother sat with me holding my hand, comforting and consoling me, assuring me that I was going to get better. My Dad found his way to my room. When he entered the room he took one look at me and his face turned pale. Gingerly he came over to my bedside. He held my hand and spoke to me quietly. Then he excused himself, not being able to see me in this condition. (He had never handled it well when someone was sick.)

Mom and Dad had to leave for a little while so they could find a hotel/motel for Dad to sleep. The nurses told Mom about a little motel on the state road. They checked in and found their way back to the hospital. She came back to my room alone. Dad couldn't do it. She patiently waited for the doctor. He finally came. She asked him "Can you tell me what is wrong with my daughter? What is going on with her?"

He responded in a very relaxed manner, "I am not sure what is wrong just yet. She is a little swollen. We are doing tests to find out where the fever is coming from and why." *A little swollen?!* That was an understatement. He then proceeded to say, "Your daughter will be fine. She will be better in twenty-four to forty-eight hours."

Mom relaxed a little after hearing those words. She thanked God this ordeal would be over soon and I would be well enough to come home. She went to the nurse's station to use the phone to call my sister Teresa and my brother Nick to give them an update. She asked them to inform Paulette of what was going on, and to try to reach my brother Sal who was driving down to Florida to vacation with his fiancée Jeanette.

Teresa and Nick decided to come up after Mom had

described my condition, and to make sure I was getting the proper care since Mom really didn't understand much of what was going on. Being a native-born Italian she had a language barrier.

Mom came back into my room. It had been a long day. She sat on the chair beside my bed. I was asleep; she was grateful for that. I'd had a very difficult day. My fever was high. I was in and out of lucidity. She sat with me quietly, remembering my beautiful face that was now marred with huge blisters. She closed her eyes as tears streamed down her face, trying to erase the vision in front of her. That night was the beginning of a vigil beside my bedside lasting the next three months.

It was a sleepless night for Mom and me. I moaned with pain throughout the night. I constantly murmured incoherent words. At other times I asked her to please help me. She didn't know what to do to ease my suffering. She was overwhelmed with her own pain and sorrow seeing me going through this. She continually comforted me; crooning stories of my childhood, holding my hand, letting me know she was by my side.

Morning came. Flowers and balloons were delivered to the room. They were from David, and Julie and Rick.

Mom was eager to speak to a doctor. The day nurses told her the doctor would be in shortly. She looked closely at me and realized the blistering was worse. I had been slightly swollen under my chin the day before but now I had a huge blister the size of a grapefruit filled with fluid. When I moved my head from side to side the huge blister would sway in the same direction. She was so afraid it was going to burst. My eyelids now had blisters the size of walnuts. I could barely open my eyes. They were small slits, and the inside of them were fiery red. I complained relentlessly how my eyes and body burned like they were on fire.

I begged over and over to please help me; the pain was unbearable. I tugged at her heartstrings. She was feeling my pain. She went to the nurse's station to get some help. She was hoping they could give me something for the pain. They told her they weren't allowed to give me anything unless the doctor ordered it.

Eventually he strolled in. He wasn't the doctor from the night before. Once again, she asked, "What is wrong with my daughter? She is getting worse before my eyes."

He answered mildly, "We are not sure what is wrong with her. We are trying to figure it out. We have to get her fever down. If we don't, she may go into a convulsive state and slip into a coma."

Mom was frustrated; she wanted answers. No one was telling her anything. It was late morning. Teresa and Nick arrived. She could hear them by the nurse's station. Teresa stepped into the room, took one look at me, and backtracked out of the room. She was horrified, unprepared for what she had seen. (It certainly wasn't what lay in bed in front of her.) The sight of me knocked the breath right out of her. She was in dismay.

I thought I heard Teresa's voice. She grabbed Nick's arm before he could go in. She tried to prepare him. I called out "Teresa is that you? Teresa, is that you? Why don't you come in to see me?" They walked in together. Nick had a look of horrific shock on his face. At that moment both their lives would be scarred forever. They would never be able to erase from their minds the image of what they just saw.

Mom hugged them both, grateful for some comfort. They stood by my bedside. My fever had not gone down.

I was in and out of delirium. Teresa was talking to me and suddenly I started to reach up to tear at my face and upper torso. Teresa held my wrists to stop me and asked me, "Why are you doing that!?"

I responded "The worms! I have to get the worms off of my face and body. Please help me! They are eating at me!" Teresa couldn't believe what she was witnessing. I was in a state of delirium. She calmed me by telling me she would take care of it. Moments later I asked Nick, "Nick, it's really hot on the beach. Can you please get me out of here?"

Nick choked a sob back and said "OK Michelle. I will get you off the beach. Is there anything else you want?"

I smiled a distorted smile and said, "Yes, can you please go to McDonalds to get me a milk shake?"

He responded, "Yes, I will go right now." They all left the room, trying to understand what was going on. They headed towards the nurse's station. Teresa and Nick demanded to have a meeting with the chief of the hospital. They were all becoming impatient and my condition was getting worse. The meeting was granted. Teresa went into the meeting herself. She was determined to express her feelings and opinions. She demanded answers. They had none. They reiterated they didn't know what was going on with me but they could assure her they were doing all they could and giving me the best care.

Teresa became inflamed. She spat, "Best care? Are you serious? My sister is in a room where the windows are open! There are flowers and balloons all over as she lays there with large open wounds!" With her body trembling with rage and tears running down her face she exclaimed, "Any idiot knows when someone has an open wound they are susceptible to infection! Your nurses are handling her with no gloves. Is that what you call best care?" Then giving her last effort she demanded, "If you don't know what is wrong with my sister I am asking you to bring a specialist in to diagnose her." They did nothing. There were no changes. Teresa's efforts were in vain.

Later that afternoon ice blankets were brought into my room. The nurses informed my mother they were using them to bring down the fever. One would be placed on the bottom and one on top. A fan was also placed beside my bed. When they placed the top ice blanket on me I screamed in pain. I begged Mom to let them take it off of me. I kept crying over and over how I was freezing. My whole entire body was trembling from the cold. She tried to calm me by telling me they would bring my fever down and I would start getting better. I cried telling her if she loved me she would ask them to remove them. She told me it was because she loved me I needed to keep them on.

She couldn't take my torture any longer. She had stayed strong until this point. She finally broke. She ran down to the family waiting room, closed the door, and screamed at the top of her lungs. Her fists were in the air asking God in Italian, "Why? Why is this happening to my daughter?" She collapsed onto the couch trying to calm herself. She turned to her faith. She did the sign of the cross and began to pray. She prayed to God for strength, courage, and her daughter's healing. This would become a ritual every moment of her days to come.

Nick and Teresa were leaving to go back home. They promised to do research on their own to find out what was happening. My mom and my dad remained. She sat in my room praying quietly. I continued to cry and whimper. There was a knock at the door, and in came David. She glared at him. It was the first time she had seen him since she got there. She imagined he was done with his weekend vacation and now heading home. His expression was sad. He looked over to me and said "Michelle, it's me, David. I'm here." I was physically incapable of responding. He looked over in Mom's direction and said to her, "Hello, Mrs. Frazzetto, how are you?"

Still glaring at him she responded, "I am angry."

He replied solemnly, "I'm sorry." He walked out of the room, and she followed. They were standing in the hallway. He repeated, "I'm sorry. I don't know what is going on."

She began to cry with frustration and anger. She lashed out at him saying, "Why is it, every time my daughter goes away with you something terrible happens to her? You are responsible for her when she is with you!" He was at a loss for words. He said nothing.

He walked back into the room and sat beside me for a while. He took my hand in his before he was ready to leave and said to me, "Michelle, you know I have to leave to go back to work. I will call you every day to see how you are doing. Hurry and get better." He then gently thumb-wrestled with me, and kissed my hand. I felt reassured. That hand gesture would be the way I knew David was with me all the days and months to follow.

Mom went down to the lobby to sit with Dad for a little while, explaining to him to the best of her ability about my condition. She also told him my brother Sal and Jeanette were heading back from Florida and coming straight to the hospital. She wasn't sure what time they would arrive. It would probably be during the early morning hours. She worried about them. When Sal had heard the news about me he had immediately turned around and headed back north without resting.

Mom came back to my room. She didn't want to miss the evening doctor. She hoped for some good news. Perhaps my fever had gone down. I had the blankets on me for five hours. The room was quiet. I seemed to be resting. She sat and began to pray. She was so lost in prayer she didn't hear the doctor walk in. Her heart quickened. She stood up and said to him, "Is her fever down? Can we take the ice blankets off?"

He frowned and replied, "No. The fever is still very high. We will have to keep the blankets on overnight."

Exasperated, she protested, "No, we can't do that. She is suffering. Please give her something for the pain."

He shook his head no and said, "We can't. If we give her something with the fever this high she may slip into a coma." He tensed slightly and continued to say, "I have to do something about the blisters on her eyelids. If I don't she may never be able to open her eyes again." He left the room and spoke with a nurse. He came back to my bed. Two nurses followed him. Each nurse firmly held down one of my arms. Mom wasn't prepared to witness what he did next. He sliced the blisters open and pressed on them so the fluid could drain. He then took his gloved finger and stuck it into my eye under my eyelid. My body thrashed with the pain. I screamed out a deep, agonizing howl. It is a sound Mom will never forget for all her living years. She collapsed into her chair holding her heart. It felt as if a stake went right through it.

Mom yelled out, "God, please help my daughter and me!"

It was another restless night for Mom and me. I pleaded with her all night to please help me and take the pain away. She just sat there with tears spilling down her face. She hurt. Her heart ached. There was her child, suffering, and there wasn't a single thing she could do. Her emotional pain was unbearable. She didn't know how much more of my suffering she could take.

The room was dark. The door opened and a stream of light came through. It caught her attention. She looked up. The nurse motioned for her to come into the hallway. The hospital guard was standing at the desk. He approached asking, "Mrs. Frazzetto, is your son Sal Frazzetto?" She nodded her head yes. He then said, "He is outside. He wanted to come in to see his sister. I told him visiting hours begin at eight o'clock and he would have to come back. He wouldn't take no for an answer. He mentioned he just drove all the way from Florida."

She looked at her watch; it was four o'clock in the morning. She asked him nicely "Would it be OK if you could let them in? If not together, maybe one at a time? They did drive from Florida. My daughter is in critical condition."

He gave her a soft smile and said, "I will let them come up one at a time." She sighed with relief. Jeanette was the first to come up. Sal stayed outside. When Sal and Jeanette had arrived they found Dad sitting under a tree crying. He had been sitting there all night waiting for Sal to arrive. Mom waited for them in the hallway.

They came into my room. Jeanette glanced at me and her entire body tensed. With a shocked expression on her face she looked at Mom and said, "What the hell happened to her? I just saw her two days ago and she was perfectly fine!" I recognized her voice. Jeanette came beside me. Stroking my hair, she spoke to me softly for a few minutes, telling me Sal was waiting to come up to see me. After a short while Sal approached the room. Jeanette tried to prepare him. The look on his face was pure devastation. Unable to speak, he lost control and began to sob.

Morning had arrived. The doctor came in. Mom didn't even have to say a word.

She could tell from his expression there was no change. He informed her the fever was still high. The ice blankets didn't work. They would be removed. He called for two nurses to come in and take them off. She stood nearby watching their every move. The first nurse rolled me on my side. When doing so, the sheet stuck to my skin. The other nurse went to pull the sheet off, and when she did, the skin of my back peeled off with the sheet.

Simultaneously Mom and I screamed aloud. My scream was blood-curdling, a sound of unbearable pain and agony. Mom's was filled with horror at what she was witnessing. Mom wanted to grab the doctor by the neck. She was irate. Her eyes flashed with anger. She began yelling. "You told me my daughter would be better in twenty-four to forty-eight hours! She is dying! I want her out of here now!"

With no expression on his face—like he has seen this on a daily basis, he responded, "She will be fine. Sometimes these things can take up to seventy-two hours."

Mom was like an animal out of its cage. She was ready to attack. And she did. With her mouth she unleashed her fury on him and said, "You must be crazy! Look at her. Her skin is not coming back in seventy-two hours. It will take months and months for her skin to grow back. I want her out of your hospital now! I refuse to allow you to kill her!" It fell on deaf ears. Once again nothing was done.

Later that morning my friend Julie came to visit me. She was horrified to see how I had declined. Knowing that I was slipping away she took the week off from work to stay by my side and advocate for me. During my lucid moments I vowed to stay strong. Julie was amazed that I had the determination to live despite my condition.

Mom and I were having a quiet afternoon. I had a few moments of clarity. We even smiled a few times. For a while it seemed like there was nothing wrong with me and she was able to overlook my blistered face and body. As I turned to look at her, the movement caused the grapefruit-sized blister under my chin to break. A torturous wail escaped my lips. Mom noticed the open wound and left the room crying for help.

A nurse, unable to ignore Mom's pain and despair anymore, took her to the side and said to her privately, "Mrs. Frazzetto, if this were my daughter, I would get her out of here. She needs to be in a burn unit in a sterile environment. They have a hot potato on their hands and they don't know what to do with it."

Mom became alarmed with what the nurse said. She hurried to a phone. Her whole body trembled with anger. When she reached my sister she cried out "Please help. They don't know what to do with your sister. They are killing her. She needs to get out of here immediately and into a hospital that has a burn unit!"

My whole family went into a panic. They tried to research my symptoms and came up with nothing. It wasn't until they mentioned to a friend of Nick what was happening that they finally had an idea of what was wrong. He vaguely remembered hearing or reading about something similar to what I was going through. He immediately started doing research. Manny found it. He gave the information to Nick and Teresa. The paper was about a condition called Stevens-Johnson Syndrome/TEN (toxic epidermal necrolysis). They were in disbelief with what they were reading. It definitely sounded like what I was going through.

Teresa immediately started to call hospitals in New York City to find out which one was equipped with a burn unit. It was Greystone Hospital. She spoke with someone in administration explaining what was happening to me. They informed her, "The hospital that she is in has to contact us before we can do anything."

Her next call was to Lakeview Hospital. She spoke with someone there. They told her "We have already contacted Greystone Hospital. There are no rooms available for your sister at this time. So there is nothing we can do."

Teresa could not believe what she was hearing. She knew they were lying. She screamed and cried with frustration as she slammed the phone down. Meanwhile my condition was deteriorating. I was slowly declining. Blisters the size of a quarter started to appear on my legs. I was hardly ever coherent.

Mom maintained her vigil beside me, praying for a miracle. The ache inside of her was consuming her. Her beautiful daughter was dying before her eyes. She felt defeated as if we had both lost the fight.

The next time she spoke with my brothers and sisters they asked all sorts of questions. They wanted to know if there was any mention of transporting me to Greystone Hospital. Mom said "No. They are doing nothing."

They became upset with her. They asked her, "Ma, are you giving up?"

She cried, "I don't know what to do. Your sister is suffering. I feel helpless."

They became enraged, urging her, "Ma, you have to fight! It's time you made some noise. You have to get her out of there. If you don't, she will die. You will bring her home and bury her." Something inside of her snapped. The thought of that reality frightened her. Those words gave her the strength and determination that she needed again.

She prepared herself for the next time the doctor came in. Once again, she was told there was no change. They were "doing everything they could" for her daughter. She lost her patience. She gave him a hard look and warned, "I want my daughter out of here! So help me God, if you don't transport her to Greystone Hospital I will put her in a car and take her back to New York City myself. If she dies on the way it will be on your conscience, but I will know I at least tried to get her help and not just let her die, lying in this hospital room!"

Mom struck a nerve. He responded quickly, "Calm down, calm down. You can't take her anywhere. She won't make it." He then informed her, "I have contacted a skin specialist from Albany to come and diagnose Michelle. He will be in tomorrow. If she needs to be transported, we will go ahead and do so."

Mom thought she was going to faint. The ringing in her ears was so loud, and her vision was blurred from all the tears. She came over to my bed. She took my hand and said "Michelle, you need to continue to fight. You are my daughter. You are strong. Tomorrow, help will come for you."

With what little strength I had left in me, I repeated, "... fight. I will fight."

The night seemed endless. Dawn arrived too slowly for the both of us. Mom sat in her chair, waiting anxiously for the specialist to come in. I was slipping away moment by moment. I just lay there. When I spoke it was nothing intelligible. Mom's anxiety grew. She began to pace throughout the room, and up and down the hallways. She looked at every man hoping he was the doctor. She came back to the room. She began to pray, holding my gold crucifix in her hands. She heard footsteps. She looked up and there he was, a doctor with a nurse beside him. She stood up and went to him.

He introduced himself. He looked over in my direction and took a deep breath. He looked over to the nurse. His expression was angry. In a stern voice he said "I can't believe you have this girl in a regular room with opened windows, flowers, and balloons. She should be in intensive care in a sterile environment."

He proceeded in a firm voice, "Get this room sterilized immediately. Get rid of the flowers and balloons. We will use the other bed to prepare her for transport. I want sterilized sheets put on the bed, and make sure you and the nurses assisting me wear sterile gowns."

He approached my bed with a sad expression. In a soft and gentle voice he said to me, "Michelle, what drugs do you take?" I responded in a barely audible voice, "I don't do any drugs."

Once again he asked "I don't mean recreational drugs. What prescriptions do you take?" I responded quietly, "Phenobarbital." The doctor stood up straighter, snapped his fingers, and said, "That is it. She is having an allergic reaction to the phenobarbital." He looked over at Mom and said, "Mom, I am going to have to ask you to leave the room. I need to prepare your daughter to be airlifted to Greystone Hospital. I have to wrap her entire body with pig skin." He then looked back at me and said, "You poor girl. I'm so sorry you have to go through this. If I was called sooner I could have helped you."

Mom left the room. She was relieved we finally got help. She called Sal to let him know they were transporting me. They came to the hospital immediately. Mom waited behind the door for some news. Her heart was racing. Her body trembled with fear. She didn't understand what was taking so long. The doctor finally came out. He approached her and said, "Mrs. Frazzetto, I'm so sorry you and your daughter have to go through this. She is ready to leave. I hope she gets better. I wish you both the best." With that, he hugged her and left.

A nurse came over to her and said "If you want to go into the room you have to gown up. She needs to be in a sterile environment."

When Mom walked into my room and looked at me, she felt like she was going to collapse. She grabbed the back of the chair to steady herself. There I lay, wrapped up like a mummy from my neck down to my feet. She couldn't believe her eyes. Her beautiful daughter was no longer recognizable.

There was a knock at the door. The nurse was summoning her to come out. They were making arrangements for transportation. We would be flown by helicopter from Lakeview Hospital to Manhattan. Mom was informed she had to pay for the helicopter up front, in full. She didn't have any money on her. She offered to pay by check or credit card. They didn't accept that. It had to be cash, money order, or certified check. She became enraged. She began hollering, "You mean to tell me if I don't have the money you won't transport my daughter?"

They responded, "We don't have a hospital helicopter. It is a private company. It has nothing to do with us."

Mom wanted to choke someone. "Were they kidding?" she shouted. "My daughter is in there dying and you are worried about money!?" She was frantic. Sal was in the lobby with Dad. She went to ask him if he had any money with him. He did not.

Sal and Jeanette went to talk to the administrator to see what they could do. They told him the same thing. Sal then offered his American Express for payment. They called the company to find out if that would be okay. They all stood there holding their breath waiting for an answer. It was a go. The American Express would do. They all let out a shriek of joy.

Mom came back to my room to give me the good news. Wiping her tears away she said, "We are finally leaving here. We are going to get you help. You have to hang in there a little longer. Keep fighting."

The nurse came in to tell Mom they were ready to leave. They told her my condition was very critical, and they weren't sure if I would survive the trip. They would have a nurse accompanying us during the flight. I was put on a stretcher. She held my hand as they were rolling me down the different hallways to the ambulance.

She was feeling very anxious. Everything was happening so rapidly. Outside, the sunlight hit her face very briefly as she made her way quickly into the ambulance. It was a short ride to the helicopter that was waiting for us. Once again we all got out and were whisked into the helicopter.

Mom took my hand and gently squeezed and kissed it. She said to me, "I love you. You are my daughter. Be strong and keep fighting."

...and even though my illness was a trial to you,
you did not treat me with contempt or scorn.
Instead you welcomed me as if I were an angel of God...

—GALATIANS 4:14

CHAPTER SEVEN

The flight seemed endless. We had finally landed at the heliport in midtown Manhattan. An ambulance waited to transport me to the hospital. I was in and out of delirium throughout the flight. All I remember is my mom continually telling me, "We are almost there," and "Be strong."

Teresa, Nick, Sal, and Jeanette were waiting at Greystone Hospital. I was immediately brought up to the burn unit. A male floor nurse expected my arrival. He spoke with the transport nurse who had accompanied me and took down all the pertinent information. They whisked me into a private room. My family members waited in the hallway.

The floor nurse came out introducing himself to all of them, wanting to know their relationship to me. He explained, "Michelle is suffering with Stevens-Johnson Syndrome, which could progress to a more life-threatening condition called TEN, also known as the syndrome of Lyell. Her physical condition is critical. We will try our best to help her. You all need to go home and get some rest. If there are any changes we will call you."

Mom stepped forward with tears in her eyes and said, "I am not going anywhere. I will stay here with my daughter. When she goes home, I will go home with her."

The nurse responded with a sad expression on his face and said, "Mama, Michelle is not going home anytime soon. It is going to take weeks and months before she leaves the hospital. What you have witnessed happening to her on the outside of her body, the same will happen to her internally. Before your daughter gets better you will see her get worse than what she is right now...if she recovers at all."

Mom's tears spilled down her face. She held her ground and replied, "I am not going home. I will stay by her side every moment. I will not leave her here by herself."

The nurse understood Mom's determination. He continued, "Michelle will be in Intensive Care. Your time with her will be very limited. You will not be able to be by her side all of the time."

She looked at him in despair. She said, "That's fine. I'm still not leaving." My sister and brothers tried to convince her to go home. They explained there was nowhere for her to sleep in the hospital. They promised to bring her to visit me every day. They lost the battle. There was no way they could convince her. She wouldn't leave me there alone as I lay there fighting for my life.

My body had declared war on itself. My condition deteriorated rapidly. A few days after arrival my kidneys began to fail. I had a terrible infection promising to shut down the kidneys as well as the rest of my body. My life was in jeopardy. I was slowly losing the battle. The nurse went looking for my mom to inform her of the change. He found her in the elevator room sitting on a little vinyl loveseat praying with her rosary. This small, six-feet-by-seven-feet area in front of the service elevator had now become her home. The nurse sat down beside her. She was startled by his presence.

He took her hands in his and spoke, "Mama, Michelle has taken a turn for the worse. She has a severe kidney infection. We can't seem to get it under control. We have given her several different types of antibiotics. None have worked. We are going to try to give her one last kind. If that doesn't work the infection will spread rampant through her body into her other organs shutting her system down. As a consequence she will die."

Mom stood up screaming and crying "No! No! No! Please I want to see her! I have to talk to her!"

The nurse gently told her, "Mama, I can't let you see her right now. She is in a very grave state. If there are any changes I will come for you. I am going to contact your children about her condition. They should come to the hospital in case Michelle doesn't make it. Mama, only God can save her now."

Mom was shaken with grief. She put her rosary around her neck and went for the elevator. Upon reaching the ground floor, she hurriedly got out, running through the hallways in despair, looking for a way out of the hospital. She was headed to St. Catherine's. Father Michael from the hospital had told her about the church. She spent her days there when she wasn't able to be by my side. With tears running down her face blurring her vision she crossed the busy streets of New York City, not caring for her own life.

She went through the church doors breathless. It was quiet inside. Her heavy breathing was the only sound. With tears streaming down her face she looked at the beautiful statue of Jesus. She walked towards it, kneeling down before it and whispered, "Lord Jesus, I have done all I can possibly do. I am now putting Michelle in your hands. Only you can save my daughter. Please Lord Jesus. I want my daughter to live. I beg you, to make her live." She knelt there for hours, crying uncontrollably. Her heart ached. Her pain was unbearable.

A priest finally came to her, touching her on her shoulder, and said gently "Ma'am, are you OK? Why are you crying? What is wrong?" My mom looked up at him with a tear-stained face.

"My daughter is in the hospital. She is in critical condition. She may not live. I asked Jesus to please save her."

The father took her hands, helping her to stand up. He responded, "Don't worry. You will see, God will answer your prayers. Grace will be given." He then guided her to the front doors and said, "Go back to the hospital, and be with your daughter. God be with you both."

Exhausted, my mother found her way back to the hospital. When she reached my floor, the nurse came running towards her yelling, "Mama, Mama, where have you been? I have been looking for you for the last hour. It's Michelle. I have news for you." My mother became alarmed not knowing what he was going to say next.

The nurse's face lit up with a smile, "I have good news... Mama, Michelle is responding to the antibiotics. Her blood work came back better." My mom let out a sob filled with relief. She dropped to her knees, praising and thanking Jesus for answering her prayers. The nurse squatted down and took her hand, inviting her, "Come Mama, I will take you in to see Michelle. We will go in there and pray with her to the Holy Spirit."

My mom's heart swelled. Her prayers had been answered. She went with the nurse into my room. They both knelt down beside my bed. Holding my hand they both began to pray for me.

...For where two or three come together in my name, there am I with them... If you believe, you will receive whatever you ask for in prayer. Matthew 18:20, 21:22

Meanwhile, Teresa and Nick, having only heard the bad news were together on their way to the hospital. As they were driving over the Brooklyn Bridge they decided to stop at St Joseph's Church to pray. The church is located on the lower east side of Manhattan. They both had attended school there. They went up the steps to the large doors of the church, hoping it was open. Neither of them recalls opening the door; it just opened on its own, and they walked in. Nick went to the left of the church to pray by the crucifixion of Christ. Teresa had gone to the right to pray by the statues of St. Teresa and St. Lucy. They were her guardian saints since her name is Maria Teresa Lucia. They both could hear one another cry across the church as they were praying. Teresa was hoping for some sort of sign that Jesus and the saints were listening to her prayers. At that very moment a priest came out from the sacristy. He noticed Teresa standing before the statues and approached her. He said "What are you doing in here?"

She was a little perplexed. She looked at him in confusion explaining, "I came in to pray for my sister. She is in the hospital. She may not live."

The priest led her to the front of the church where Nick had joined them. The priest then asked a little confused himself, "What door did you come in from?" Teresa and Nick were befuddled. They were not sure why he was asking that question. The answer should have been obvious to the priest. They pointed at the front door they walked through. They were both in disbelief with what they saw. The door had a large lock with a chain on the handles. The priest looked at their shocked faces, saying, "If you came in through that door to pray, your prayers will then be answered."

The priest escorted them to the door, unlocking it. They both left feeling dazed. They didn't understand nor did they have any answers for what just happened. They hoped it was a good sign. It was a surreal experience for the both of them.

They arrived at the hospital. Their feelings were running wild. They didn't know what to expect once they got to my floor. They walked out of the elevator, and there sat Mom. She looked up and went to them. She said "Michelle is out of danger. She is responding to the antibiotics. She is doing better." They all hugged each other crying with joy. Teresa and Nick looked at each other in wonder. At that moment they believed there had been a divine intervention.

Mom thought the worst was over. It was only the beginning. My diagnosis had changed from SJS (Stevens Johnson Syndrome) to TEN (Toxic Epidermal Necrolysis.) While I recovered from the kidney infection the blistering progressed in a fierce way. Blisters had formed on ninety percent of my body. They were all over my arms, hands, upper torso, legs, feet, and spreading to my scalp. More blisters appeared on my face, disfiguring me further. The only area on my body that didn't have any blisters was my abdomen. My beautiful hair was falling out in clumps. I lay there naked. Silver sulfadiazine patches were placed over my open wounds. My entire body oozed blood and clear fluids. A bed sheet was tented over a stack of pillows that surrounded me, careful not to touch my bleeding body and allowing me to maintain some sort of dignity. They had sedated me so I wouldn't feel the pain of what I was going through. I had very few episodes of lucidity during this time. The nurses came in hourly to change my bed sheets. The blood and fluid would saturate them quickly. Mom assisted them whenever she was able. She made me little pads with gauze and cotton to cushion the mask and straps of the oxygen mask. They were digging into my ears and nose, threatening to deform them.

Each morning there was a large lump of dried blood sealing my lips together. Mom would come in each day, placing ice on my lips, softening the blood to separate them. She did this so she could swab the inside of my mouth, removing the sloughed-off mucous membranes that were making me gag, and cleaning the bleeding gums to prevent losing my teeth. The nurses were grateful for Mom's helping hand.

The time came where they had to shave my hair off. The blisters had spread further into my scalp. They were concerned I would get another infection, penetrating the skull, possibly causing brain damage. It was a daily battle for me and Mom both. With every change that occurred with my body, Mom remained strong. She constantly had an ache in her heart for all my pain and suffering. She found comfort in her faith. The nurses embraced her with open arms. They had become her family. Little children, who were in the hospital for burns, gravitated to her kindness.

The hospital had now become her home, and the staff and patients were now her family. She slept on the little vinyl love-seat in the elevator room. She bathed in the public bathroom. Housekeepers befriended her. They all felt her pain. They tried to make her comfortable by giving her pillows, sheets, and towels. When there was an extra tray of food, the nurses would give it to her. They all admired the strength and love she had for me. Her only contact with the outside world was going to church and receiving visits from my family. Nick, Glenda and the boys would come every night bringing Mom dinner each time they came.

David also came every night after work. David remained dedicated to me. He came for a couple of hours sitting at my bedside, or at Mom's little area talking with her. Everyone I loved and knew was going through internal turmoil. They were all hoping and praying I would make it through this alive.

The first week passed. My condition was still very critical. I was losing weight rapidly due to the open wounds that were losing blood and fluids. Weighing me each day was imperative. (When my weight loss stopped it would be an indication to them the disease had finished manifesting.) They weighed me like they would an animal. Straps were put underneath me, lifting my body onto a metal scale. They needed to be extremely careful not to tear open my blistered skin. This was not a simple task for them. By the second week I had lost a startling twenty pounds.

Later in the week my hands swelled up like two balloons. (They were hoping this wasn't going to happen.) It would mean I would have to have a procedure done exposing another area susceptible to infection. Mom looked up when she saw one of her favorite nurses walk into the room. The nurse was tall, slim, and blonde. She reminded Mom of me. She sat beside Mom and said, "Mama, I am going to have to do a procedure on Michelle's hands. There is too much fluid in them to wait for it to absorb. I'm going to take her across the hall to a sterile room. I will let you know when it is over."

Mom looked into the nurse's beautiful blue eyes and said, "I want to be there with Michelle. The sound of my voice will reassure her. Please allow me to come in with her."

The nurse didn't want to argue with Mom. She gently said, "Mama, I don't think that is a good idea. You won't be able to handle what I'm about to do."

Mom straightened her back and squeezed the nurse's hand and pleaded, "Please, I am strong. I need to be there for Michelle."

The nurse stood up and with admiration on her face she said, "Go and get scrubbed up. Someone will come for you." Mom walked into the plain, white sterile room. There was a little sink to the left of the door, and a large window allowing sunshine to fill the room. The nurse approached. "Mama I need for you to stand to the right by the door as I work on Michelle's left hand. When I'm done with the left hand, we will switch places, and you can stand by the window so I can work on her right hand."

Mom looked at her and nodded. The nurse was preparing her instruments. Mom had no idea what the nurse was going to do and she wasn't prepared to witness what was about to happen. The nurse was ready to begin. She looked at Mom and said "Are you ready Mama?"

Mom held her breath and once again nodded her head. The nurse picked up a scalpel and made a little incision on the top of my hand by the wrist. She then reached for the surgical scissors and began to cut the skin around my entire wrist. Placing the scissors down the nurse took my hand in hers and began to peel off the skin from my hand as if it was a glove. The fluid splattered everywhere. My hand was like a piece of raw meat. Mom was horrified. She immediately looked over at me to see if I was feeling the pain. She became unsteady on her feet. She lost all color in her face. She thought she was going to faint.

The nurse looked up at her and said, "Mama. Mama, are you alright?" Mom was holding her breath. She couldn't speak. Tears spilled down her beautiful face under her mask. She finally found her voice and said, "I'm alright. I'm strong." The response was more to convince herself rather than the nurse. They switched spots. The same procedure was done to my other hand. When it was over the nurse put silver sulfadiazine patches on my fingers and hands, then wrapped them with gauze. Mom was in utter shock. She couldn't believe what she had just witnessed. Inwardly she thought: What in God's name is happening to my beautiful daughter?

Mom took the skin with my beautiful long nails still attached over to the sink, washed it clean and placed it in a sterile bag. The nurse sadly noticed what she was doing but she didn't stop her. She fully understood the reason why. It was like something snapped in Mom's head and a piece of her heart was torn out of her chest. She would not allow them to throw away a part of me in the trash as if I was nothing but a piece of garbage. Tears streamed down her face as Mom left the room holding the bag in her hand. She was devastated by what she had just seen and the pain was too much for her to bear. Her only thought was of my beautiful nails. They would be the only part she had left of me should I die.

Several days later the bottom of my feet began to swell. The doctors wanted to stop the progression of the blisters. It was important the same situation did not occur as on my hands. Removing the skin from both my feet was not an option. The skin of the feet takes longer to heal because of its thickness. It would be another open wound possibly allowing another area to get an infection. In addition, there was a greater possibility of my feet healing deformed, prohibiting me from ever being able to walk again. In the end, they put on braces that looked like little booties. The booties would compress the blisters allowing the body to absorb the liquid and prevent the feet from filling further with fluid. It also separated each of my toes and forced my feet to form an arch. Each bootie was extremely uncomfortable. In my lucid moments I would plead with my mom to please have the nurses remove them from my feet. Mom would reply in a sad voice, "Michelle, they have to stay on for your own good."

I would cry with pain and say, "If you love me, you will have them take them off."

Broken-hearted she would patiently respond, "Michelle, it is because I love you they need to stay on. One day you will thank me when you are walking in your beautiful high heels again."

It was still a very long road ahead for Mom and me. Days passed and the disease continued to manifest. Mom still lived in the elevator room refusing to go home. Her vigil continued by my bedside. The nurses became concerned with her well-being. Mom wasn't eating and sleeping properly. She had no regard for herself. It was becoming visually apparent to everyone.

One day a nurse approached her when she was sitting in my room. The nurses had the utmost respect for my Mom. They had grown to love her. The nurse placed her hand on Mom's shoulder. Mom looked up at her anxiously thinking the nurse was going to ask her to leave because her time was up. The nurse sat next to Mom and said, "Mama, I am working the night shift this evening. I will be Michelle's nurse. Why don't you go and sleep in my dorm tonight. You can get a good night's sleep and tomorrow you can take a real shower." Mom hung her head down. She was exhausted. With tear-filled eyes she looked back at the nurse. The nurse understood her dilemma and continued, "Mama, you are not going to be any good for Michelle if you get sick. It's only one night. She will be OK, I promise." Mom relented and nodded her head as tears spilled down her face. The nurse took her hands and said "I will allow you to stay longer to visit tonight. When you are ready, come and get me for the key." Mom stayed with me as long as she possibly could. She felt guilty leaving me. Holding my bandaged hand she explained to me where she was going for the night and she would be back in the morning.

The next day Mom was eager to see me. She was hoping for an overnight miracle but there was none. My condition was still very critical. I lay there semi-conscious, still fighting for my life. There were a few moments of consciousness throughout the day. During those times, I could hear Mom praying or just talking to me always encouraging me to get better. I could feel her love and strength pour into me.

Other days I seemed to be more aware of my surroundings. I would ask about my family, and David. One day I had a strong desire to see my dad. Subconsciously I knew he had not been in to see me and that hurt me. Teresa and Nick came to visit me later that day. I begged them to ask Dad to come to see me. They called and pleaded with him to come to the hospital. With much reluctance he did, knowing he would make me extremely happy. They were all in the hallway. Dad hesitated at the door. He was nervous, not knowing what to expect. The last time he had seen me, my face was marred with blisters. Teresa and Nick tried to prepare Dad beforehand explaining my appearance. They both urged him to go into my room. He walked in. Teresa and Nick followed behind. He saw Mom sitting on the chair by my bed. He had not seen her in two weeks. He didn't have the courage to look my way. Never averting his eyes from her he said, "Paolina." Mom turned in her chair and looked at him. She had tears in her eyes. She was happy to see him.

When I heard his voice I called out to him, "Papa, you're here." He looked in my direction and froze. His heart split in two. He couldn't believe his eyes. All he saw were tubes and wires hooked up to me. My face was unrecognizable. It was raw skin covered with ointment. The only recognizable thing about me was my voice. He was stunned.

In a choked voice, he managed to answer, "Ciao Michelle. I'm here." Unsteady on his feet he grabbed the foot rail. He began to sweat and his face turned pale. He looked at Nick in a panic as his legs gave out. Nick reached out for him before he hit the floor, placing him on the chair. I was scared and upset. I didn't know what all the commotion was about. Teresa went to get a nurse. The nurse came in with a wheelchair taking my dad to the Emergency Room. Mom left to go with Dad. Teresa and Nick stayed with me trying to calm me down. The nurse came in, increased my sedative, and all went black. The next time I saw my dad was when I went home three months later.

It was the first week in August. With much trepidation, Teresa was preparing to go back to Italy. She didn't know if I was going to survive what was happening to me. For all she knew it might be the last time she saw me alive. With a heavy heart she said goodbye to me. She promised to call the hospital to see how I was doing. My mind was jumbled. I didn't understand everyone's sorrow. I didn't grasp the severity of what was happening to me. My condition remained unchanged for a few days. Everyone thought the nightmare was over. It was the calm before the storm.

Once again I took another turn for the worse. One evening I was having difficulty breathing. Mom noticed my breathing had become shallow. I was gasping for air. She brought it to the nurse's attention. The nurse looked at a monitor for my oxygen levels. They seemed to be low but she wasn't too concerned about it. She showed Mom what to look for. She explained if it got too low the alarms would go off, and at that point they would put me on a respirator. Mom stared at the monitor, holding my hand, praying for that not to happen. Mom's visiting time was up. She didn't want to leave me just yet. Her voice seemed to calm my breathing. She decided to try to outsmart the nurses. She closed the curtain around the bed and then she sat with her legs beneath her in the chair so they wouldn't see her feet. She hoped they would think she had left. Mom told me what she was doing and I giggled (a sound that now was so foreign to both our ears.)

I informed Mom I didn't want them to give me a tracheotomy for any reason. I refused to live that way. I would prefer to die. I asked Mom to promise me. She did with much hesitation. She understood why I was saying that. My grandmother had one. It was the most awful thing. I remembered her coughing things out of the opening in her throat. In order to speak she had to put a plug in it. It wasn't something I wanted to live with. The nurse finally came in to check on me. Mom was caught. She had fallen asleep with her head on the bed, holding my hand. The nurses had empathy for Mom for all she was going through. The nurse woke her gently, asking her to leave. Mom took my hand and kissed it and said, "I love you. I will see you in the morning."

I responded softly "I love you too." They would be the last words I spoke to Mom in a very long time. During the night my breathing became labored. I gasped for air. My chest felt as if I had a ton of bricks on it. My lungs hurt. Nurses were coming in and out of my room in a hurry. Monitor alarms were going off in all directions. I panicked. I didn't know what was happening to me. I was trying to listen for Mom's voice. She wasn't in the room. My anxiety mounted. I tried to scream out but I couldn't. I was having difficulty catching my breath. A nurse saw me struggling trying to say something. She came over to my bedside. Trying to calm me she said, "Michelle, I am going to give you some medicine to sedate you. You are going to be fine, Babygirl. Just relax and close your eyes." Those were the last words I heard.

The following morning Mom came in to see me. She was shocked when she saw me hooked up to a respirator. She ran over to my bedside and tried to talk to me. I couldn't respond because I had been intubated during the night. Mom was hoping by the sound of her voice I would open my eyes. I didn't. Mom pleaded with me, "Michelle, if you can hear my voice, squeeze my hand." I did nothing. I could hear her voice. I desperately wanted to respond, but my body betrayed me. She became alarmed. She ran out of my room looking for the nurse who was in charge of me. She found her at the nurse's station. "What happened to Michelle last night?"

The nurse looked at Mom sadly and said, "Mama, I don't know. We just changed shifts. I will look in her chart and let you know. Meet me in Michelle's room." Mom sat patiently waiting for the nurse as tears trickled down her face. She didn't understand what could have happened to me during the night. She was lost in thought when the nurse came in. The nurse pulled a chair next to Mom's and sat down, gathering her strength. She dreaded giving Mom the bad news. She had become so fond of Mom she didn't have the courage to break her heart further. The nurse held both of Mom's hands and looked into her beautiful brown eyes saying, "Mama, Michelle had a very difficult night. You know she was having trouble breathing. It isn't her lungs but her heart. Michelle's heart is extremely weak. It isn't pumping hard enough to get oxygen throughout her body. Putting her on the respirator will help the heart so it doesn't have to work so hard."

Mom leaned back into the chair, closed her eyes, and began to cry. She couldn't believe all the suffering I was going through. The nurse knelt in front of Mom and hugged her. Wiping a tear off Mom's face she said, "Mama, we told you when Michelle first came in she was going to get worse before getting better. This situation is very critical. If her heart fails she will go into cardiac arrest and we are not sure she will make it through that. Her body is just too weak." Mom let out heart-wrenching sobs. In anger she began to punch the arm of the chair, crying out "No! No! No! This can't be happening to my beautiful daughter!"

The nurse hugged Mom tighter, trying to calm her down. Tears filled the nurse's eyes, feeling Mom's agony. Comforting her, the nurse said softly, "Mama, all of us are praying for Michelle. Patients, family members of the patients, doctors, staff, everyone, it seems like the entire hospital, and we are going to bombard the heavens for Michelle's recovery. You and Michelle have captured our hearts."

Allowing the words to console her, Mom slumped in the chair with exhaustion. She looked at the nurse asking, "Why can't Michelle hear me or answer me?"

The nurse answered gently, "We had to put her in a medically-induced coma. She will be more comfortable this way.

Her body is in distress. This will be easier for her." Rubbing Mom's hands, the nurse proceeded by saying, "Mama, if you want to go home and get some rest that wouldn't be a bad idea for you. Michelle doesn't know if you are here or not."

Mom sat up in her chair and said "No. I will not leave her here alone. My place is here by her side."

The nurse nodded her head solemnly and said, "I understand, Mama."

Two days later my heart began to decline. The heart wasn't receiving the proper nutrients from my body or the intravenous tube. As a consequence it was becoming weaker and weaker by the moment. The doctors wanted to do a procedure called TPN (total parenteral nutrition.) They had to place a catheter into a main blood vessel. The tip of the catheter goes into the right atrium, a chamber of the heart. The nutrition then goes into the body through the catheter, entering the blood stream. This procedure will allow the body and heart to absorb the nutrients quicker.

The doctors had two problems. The first problem was trying to find an area of skin to place the catheter. The other problem was health insurance didn't pay for the bag of nutrients. Each bag cost from seven hundred dollars to one thousand dollars per twenty-four hours.

The doctors and nurses had a meeting with Mom letting her know the gravity of my situation and what they would like to do. The room for the meeting was small. It held a conference table which sat six people. Two doctors and two head nurses were talking with each other. When Mom sat down, all their attention was directed to her. One doctor looked at Mom straight on and said, "Mrs. Frazzetto, we all have come to an agreement in regards to how we would like to proceed with Michelle's care. The head nurses have informed you of Michelle's current situation with her heart. Is that correct?"

Mom looked at him sadly and said, "I don't understand much, but yes they have told me."

The doctor's demeanor softened a little. He said, "We would like to place a feeding line called TPN. This will help strengthen Michelle's heart, giving her a greater chance of survival." Mom looked down at her hands. Tears began to pool in her eyes. The doctor proceeded, "There are two problems. Michelle doesn't have a lot of skin left on her body in order to place the TPN, and the other problem is we are not sure if her insurance will cover it. In case her insurance won't pay for it, are you willing to cover the cost? It is very expensive and she will need at least seven to ten days of it."

Mom stared at him incredulously. She could not believe how money came before human life. She answered firmly, "Yes, I will pay anything to save my daughter."

The doctor nodded his head and said, "We will check with the insurance first and let you know. The only area we can put the TPN at this point is in her neck. Normally the catheter could stay in, but in her case because of the sloughing of her skin it will have to be put in different spots in the neck." He continued and as he was preparing to end the meeting he said, "An x-ray will be taken every time a new catheter is placed to make sure it is positioned in the right atrium. This will mean a lot of exposure to radiation. Do you understand?"

Mom's tears trickled down her cheeks. "Yes, I understand." Mom sat there and cried, wondering if she made the right decision, as everyone exited the room except for the head nurse, a man whom she had nicknamed White Angel. (Mom had given him that name because when he ran up and down the hallway his feet didn't look like they were touching the floor and his white lab coat spread open like wings reminding her of an angel. He had an angelic way about him.) He sat next to Mom and held her hands as he said, "Mama, we are waiting for the insurance company to call us back. I will let you know what the outcome is. Why don't we go to Michelle's room and pray with her."

Several hours had passed since the meeting. Mom was sitting in her little elevator room talking and reading to Jon-Pierre (one of the burn children who had become extremely close to my family) when "White Angel" came running down the hallway, calling out, "Mama, we just got the OK from Michelle's insurance! Michelle is a lucky girl. They are willing to pay for whatever she needs."

Mom was so excited by the news she reached for Jon-Pierre and hugged him, telling him, "One day my little girl is going to be well just like you."

The boy looked up at her smiling, and said, "Mama, I am happy for you and your daughter. I can't wait to meet your little girl."

They were going to attempt to put in the first TPN. Mom wasn't allowed in the room when they did this procedure. She stood behind my door holding her breath, peering through the little glass window watching what everyone was doing. The nurse finally came out letting her know it was successful. Mom thanked God and released a sigh of relief. They allowed her to come in and see me for a few minutes. She approached my bed thinking so much had changed in the last twenty-four hours. I had a tube in my throat, a catheter in my neck, and intravenous tubes wherever they could be placed.

Mom brought a chair beside my bed. She began to talk to me quietly. I could hear her and I was comforted by her voice. She repeated over and over, "Michelle you are my daughter. You are strong like me. You need to fight."

I could hear her cry. I wanted to reach out and comfort her. I wanted to tell her I was okay. I didn't understand why she was crying. I couldn't move and speak. In my head I thought it was the oddest thing. Why can't I reach for her? Why can't I talk? My heart ached for my mom. I needed for her to stop crying. I could do nothing. I was helpless. The nurse came in letting her know it was time for her to go. She took my bandaged hand and gently kissed it and said, "I love you and I will see you later."

I was going to receive my third bag of nutrients. Once again another catheter had to be placed into my right atrium. It was becoming more and more difficult to find a spot in my neck to put the line in. It seemed as if all was going smoothly on this particular day until the alarms went off on the heart and respiratory monitors. Everyone in the room began to scramble. Orders were being barked for an x-ray. I was having trouble breathing. I felt like I was suffocating. I was frightened. I didn't know what was going on. Was I going to die?

Mom was observing all of this through the little window on the door. She was stricken. Panic crept up her spine. She knew something was terribly wrong. Staff was running in and out of my room bringing equipment and machines. She knew better not to ask any questions. She got on her knees beside the door and began to pray. It seemed like a lifetime before a nurse came to her. The nurse squatted in front of her and rubbed her arm letting Mom know she was there. Mom opened her eyes and looked at the nurse anxiously trying to read the nurse's expression. The nurse gave Mom a slight smile and helped her to her feet. She said "Mama, come with me, and I will tell you what happened."

Mom reached for the nurse's hand and said "Is Michelle OK?"

The nurse nodded and said "Yes. Let's go and talk." Before Mom followed, she peeked through the little window to make sure I was OK. The nurse brought Mom to the little conference room. They sat, and the nurse took Mom's hands in hers saying, "Michelle is critical but stable. When the doctor tried to put the catheter in, it went in the wrong direction puncturing her left lung. We had to make an incision on her left side so we could put a tube into the lung to keep it inflated. She is comfortable, Mama. We are doing our best for her."

Mom's tears were streaming down her face. She couldn't believe what she was hearing. She closed her eyes and thought to herself, how much suffering can one person endure? Mom was going through the emotional suffering. I was going through the physical suffering.

Pictures at Greystone Hospital

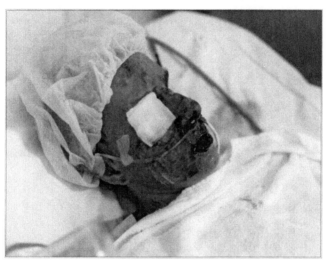

Head - Eyes - Lips

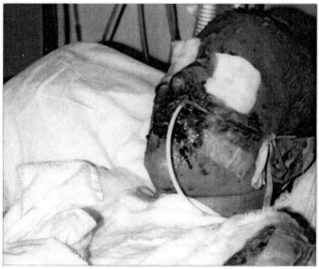

Breathing Tube - Nose - Ears

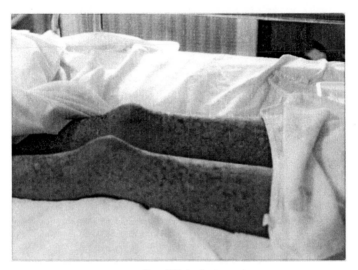

Leg Blistering

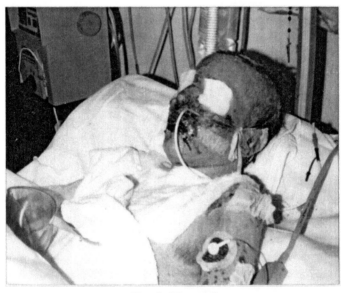

Hands Wrapped

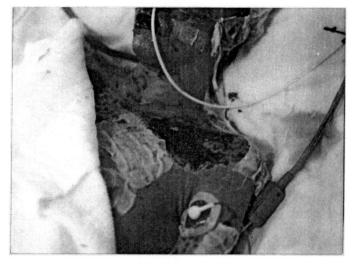

Upper Body

This day...I have set before you life and death
...now choose life...
DEUTERONOMY 30:19

CHAPTER EIGHT

Hours turned into days; days turned into weeks. My condition still had not changed. Mom still lived in the elevator room, never leaving to go home. She established a routine. Every morning when she came in to see me she opened the shades letting the daylight in. She would then tell me the date and how the weather was outside. She also described in detail what she was wearing each day. She wasn't sure if I could hear her talking to me but she did it anyway. The nurses told her it was wonderful she was doing that because it was a form of therapy. It would keep my mind alert and active. Incredibly I could hear everything she was telling me. Mom also had them turn on the TV in my room. She left it on when she wasn't there. I was able to follow a soap opera and listen to *The Preppy Murder*. Mom had placed pictures of me on the wall behind my bed so everyone could see what I looked like before this happened to me.

Sal and Jeannette would come once a week. Sal was a truck driver. He was out of town during the week, so they would come on the weekends. Nick, Glenda and the boys would come every night bringing Mom dinner and a change of clothing. Not everyone could come in to see me at one time. When Nick was waiting in the hallway he would let the boys play with Jon-Pierre. Sometimes Nick would put Jon-Pierre in a wheelchair and race through the hallways, bringing a little fun and laughter into his life. He had burned in a house fire. His mom was also in the hospital. Jon-Pierre's entire body was burned except for his private area and his beautiful face.

Teresa would call the hospital from Italy every few days. If the nurses weren't busy they would bring the phone to my ear, hoping I could hear her voice. David still came every night after work and on the weekends. Stacie came to see me whenever she had a chance. She was busy with her new life, and a baby. Everyone remained strong, willing all their strength into me. They were all praying and hoping for a change in my condition soon. I remained comfortably numb. It wasn't all of the time I could hear what was happening around me. It seemed as if my mind was a blur. I drifted in and out of consciousness.

During this period of time I had a divine experience as well as a look into the abyss. As I lay there in my coma I had a vision of Jesus. I was walking along a path. It was very bright and serene. White fine mist surrounded me. It was like walking through clouds except for what I was walking towards. I could see someone in the distance and I wanted to reach them. I couldn't determine if it was a man or a woman. As I walked closer I could see the person was in a kneeling position wearing something white. The hands were clasped together upon a huge rock. The figure seemed to be praying. I didn't want to create a disturbance so I was careful not to make any noise. As I got closer I realized it was a man. I could only see his profile. His head was slightly positioned up like he was talking to someone. My heart quickened. I recognized this man. It was Jesus. I began to walk faster towards him. He turned to look at me. He immediately held his hand up to stop me from coming forward. I abruptly stopped. Looking at him in confusion I said, "Why are you stopping me? I want to be with you." His expression was gentle.

When he finally spoke, he said, "Michelle, it is not your time. You need to go back to your mother." I stood there and cried. Why was he turning me away? As quickly as that scene appeared it vanished.

My other experience wasn't as pleasant. I was in front of my house trying to unlock the front door. The keys didn't fit the lock. I was perplexed. I looked at the key to see if I had the correct one. And I did. I rang the doorbell. Mom was supposed to be at home but there was no answer. I went around the side of the house, heading towards the back to see if there was a door unlocked. Maybe Mom was hanging wash on the clothes line. As I approached the back yard I noticed this huge crater in the earth. It frightened me. I tentatively walked closer towards the edge of the pit. I could hear loud voices and laughter coming from below. I was astounded with what I witnessed. There were people in the hole. They were doing incomprehensible things. People were having orgies. They were drinking alcohol out of fountains. Everyone's face was distorted. I was in disbelief. As I stood there I felt a presence to my left. I looked over to see who it was. A man dressed in a black suit stood several feet away from me. I looked at his face to see if I would recognize him. I didn't. He was a fairly good looking man. I asked him, "Who are you?" He smiled and his face became contorted. It was like he was snarling at me. His smile exuded pure evilness. A chill ran down my spine.

I realized who he was. It frightened me. He sensed my terror and he began to laugh louder and louder. I wanted to run but couldn't. I was frozen in place. Suddenly, out of nowhere, a strong rush of wind blew through. Three angels grabbed me lifting me off the ground, sweeping me away. I didn't know what was happening to me. The angels placed me inside my house at the bottom of the stairway. Mom waited for me on the top of the landing holding a bouquet of roses. I looked up at her and began to crawl up the steps to try to reach her. I felt sick and extremely fatigued. Every step I crawled up seemed to take an eternity. I had no strength. I cried with pain. I was vomiting convulsively. Mom was saying "Michelle, I know it is hard for you. If you don't want to fight anymore, I understand."

I thought to myself, *why is she saying that*? It made me more determined to keep going. Mom looked down at me, tears streaming down her face. She knew she couldn't help me. It was something I had to do myself.

Once again she said, "Michelle, you are so sick. If you want to give up, you can. It is OK." Anger flared through me.

I cried back, "I will not give up! I will continue to fight!" A few more steps before I could reach her I extended my arm so she could help me up the rest of the way. Mom grasped my hand in a strong grip and pulled me into her arms. She cradled me like a baby.

Stroking my hair she reassured, "I love you. I will be here every step of the way to help you." Looking at it twenty-eight years later, it is still vivid in my mind. I knew then I had the freedom to choose whether I wanted to continue to fight and live, or give up and die.

I was given a total of ten bags of nutrients. It stabilized my condition. My heart was no longer as weak as it was. That was a big step forward in my recovery. Nurses still came in every two hours to change my bandages. Doctors did their rounds with medical students. It was an educational experience for them to see a patient with TEN. It was such a rare occurrence, one or two in a million. They would only read about it in medical textbooks. When medical and nursing students came into my room Mom was on high alert. She was nervous about them not having the experience to take care of me. She would stand behind my door, peering through the little window, watching them like a hawk.

One day two students came into my room. They had to draw blood. Mom watched them. They were beside my bed looking at my arm for a vein. The first student inserted the needle three times and was unsuccessful. The other student wanted to try to find the vein. They were both laughing, motioning with their hands who would be able to get it. The second one tried several times and was unsuccessful as well. They were exiting my room laughing and joking around as I lay there with blood trickling down my arm. Mom couldn't believe her eyes. There was blood all over the sheets. As they came through the door, Mom lashed out at them, saying "You left my daughter laying there bleeding!" She launched forward reaching for his throat. Grabbing his shirt she said, "What do you think she is, an animal? You didn't even bother to put a Band-Aid on her."

The student pushed her away, telling her "Lady, you are crazy." All shook up, he yelled for a nurse at the nurse's station. One came running over. The student said to the nurse, "This lady is crazy. She just tried to attack me."

Mom launched towards him again. The nurse grabbed her. She tried to struggle out of the nurse's grip and said, "Yes! I am crazy. She is my daughter. She is not your sacrificial lamb!"

The nurse held Mom and said "Mama Frazzetto, please calm down." Mom's body shook with rage. She remained in the nurse's embrace and began to cry. Angrily she said, "I won't allow anyone to mistreat my daughter."

Five weeks had passed since the nightmare began. It was my fourth week in the Burn Unit of Intensive Care. Up until this point I had a private room. Since my condition had somewhat stabilized they now put me in a different room in Intensive Care where it could be shared with other critical patients.

Mom one afternoon was heading back to her elevator room. She had been busy with Jon-Pierre that morning. They had put a compression garment on his entire body to help with scarring. Little Jon-Pierre was having trouble feeding himself so Mom volunteered to help out. As Mom walked down the hallway, she looked at her watch. She hoped it was time for visiting hours. Not too far from my door, she noticed a lady standing there crying. She went over to her inquiring, "Hello Miss, why are you crying?"

The lady looked up at Mom and said, "My son is a fireman. He was putting out a fire in an apartment building and got burned."

Mom gave her a hug for encouragement. When she released her she said, "Is he burned badly?"

The woman wiped her tears answering, "Both of his arms, his chest, neck, and part of his face."

Mom felt her pain. She knew what this woman was going through.

Mom then asked, "What room is your son in?" The woman pointed to a door. Mom was surprised. It was my room. Mom looked at the lady and said, "My daughter is in the same room. We have been here for four weeks."

The woman looked at Mom sympathetically and said, "I saw someone in the other bed. She was unrecognizable with all the bandages. I didn't know if the person was a girl or a boy."

Mom took the woman's hands. "Are you religious?"

The woman answered, "Yes."

Mom then said, "Visiting hours are not for a little while. I am going to church. Would you like to come with me?"

The woman was surprised at my mother's warm-heartedness. She responded, "I would love to but I can't. I am waiting for the doctors to let me know how my son is doing."

Mom understood completely. She said, "I am sure we will see each other again. I will pray for your son."

The woman responded, "And I will pray for your daughter."

Mom left to go to church. Walking down the hallway she thought to herself, "I understand the pain this woman has in her heart for her son."

The following afternoon the woman saw Mom sitting in the elevator room. She sat beside Mom and said, "I brought you something. It is a newsletter, and holy oil from a saint who has done a lot of miracles." Mom was touched by this woman's kindness. She took the holy oil and newsletter and began to read.

Mom asked her, "Who is this saint?"

The woman responded, "I am Greek. This saint is a Greek saint. Her name is St. Irene Chrisovalantou. I truly believe in this saint. She has answered many of my prayers."

Mom was intrigued. She was eager to read the newsletter. She looked at the woman, held her hand, and said, "Thank you so much for this. I will pray to St. Irene for my daughter and for your son." They hugged one another as tears trickled down their cheeks.

In the next several weeks my condition improved. The blistering stopped. They were able to keep my fever down. I was no longer losing so many fluids. My weight had stabilized. I had lost a total of forty-five pounds. I now weighed seventy-three pounds, down from one hundred eighteen. I was still deeply sedated but with more episodes of lucidity. Even though I was still intubated, Mom came in every morning to talk to me.

One day Mom said to me, "Michelle, it is the last week in August. September is approaching soon and the weather is going to get cooler. I am not sure I can stay here when it gets cold." In my fuzzy mind I thought: What is she saying? August? September? How long have I been in here? Where am I? I was frightened and confused. I wasn't sure what was going on with me. I wanted to communicate with Mom to get answers. Mom could tell I was trying to say something. I began to get agitated. I couldn't talk. I tried to move my fingers so I could spell out words. Mom didn't understand. We were both frustrated. I cried. Tears spilled down my face. Mom wiped them and said, "I will think of something so you and I can communicate. I promise."

Mom kept her promise. The following day she came in with a magic slate. It was a square piece of cardboard with a waxy black coating. It had a plastic sheet of paper on top. It came with a small writing tool. When you wrote words, the translucent top sheet revealed the letters impressed into the black coating. When you peeled the plastic sheet up, the words would disappear. It was difficult for me to hold on to the writing tool. My hands were still bandaged. Mom helped me to hold it. After I wrote a few letters of a word Mom would try to guess what the word was so I didn't have to spell the entire word. I would nod or shake my head yes or no if she guessed right or wrong.

When I wanted to write a new word, I would move my hand like I was erasing a blackboard. This is how we communicated for weeks when I had my brief moments of coherency.

It was during this period of time the doctors had another meeting with Mom. My respirator needed to be removed to prevent any infection. Once again everyone gathered in the conference room. The doctor looked at Mom and said, "Mrs. Frazzetto, I am going to go over all of Michelle's progress with you." Mom looked at him in surprise. Her heart leaped into her throat. The doctor continued, "Michelle has shown some improvements in certain areas and in others she is still struggling. We need to remove Michelle from the respirator sometime this week. She has been on it for the maximum length of time possible. She is at risk of infection. If that happens, it will jeopardize her progression." Mom became anxious. She remained quiet and wondered to herself what would happen at the moment they took me off the respirator. Her answer came immediately. The doctor cleared his throat and proceeded "Once we remove the respirator, if Michelle is not able to breathe on her own, we will have to give her a tracheotomy."

Mom looked up in alarm and protested, "No. Michelle and I have discussed that possibility and she refuses to have a tracheotomy done."

The doctor looked at Mom solemnly advising, "Don't make any decisions just yet. Let us take it off and see what will happen."

There was a loud roar in her ears. She couldn't hear anything else the doctor was saying. She stared at him blankly. The only thought going through her mind was the promise she had made to me. She promised not to allow them to give me a tracheotomy. Tears trickled down her face. She was confused.

She didn't want me to resent her for the rest of my life for betraying my trust. On the flip side she couldn't let me die. She didn't know what to do. The doctor gained her attention once again when he said, "If all goes well. We will start removing some of Michelle's bandages. A small layer of skin is starting to grow back. That is great news." Mom gave him a faint smile. Her heart remained troubled about the respirator. With those last words said, the meeting was over.

Later that evening, Mom had a great desire to be by my side. Visiting hours were over. She decided she would sneak into my room. She looked down the hallway towards the nurse's station. No one was there. Taking her sneakers off, she quietly walked further toward my room. She stopped briefly by the door of the nurse's lounge. She peeked in. All the nurses were busy talking and drinking coffee. She ran quickly past that doorway and proceeded to my room. She came beside my bed, took my hand, and kissed it. It woke me up. I heard Mom whisper, "Michelle, it's me. I'm not supposed to be here, but I wanted to pray with you." I nodded my head. She closed the curtain and sat on the chair whispering, "I have some holy oil from St. Irene. I am going to put a little bit all over your body, especially over your lungs. Michelle, you have to have faith and believe you will be healed."

Once again I nodded my head. Praying, Mom took the oil and began to dab it all over my body. Mom was so engrossed in prayer she didn't hear the nurse come in. When he pulled back the curtain, he saw Mom holding my hand and her head bowed. He began to say something and abruptly stopped. He realized she was praying with me. He took a step back and closed the curtain. He left the both of us to our prayers. Fifteen minutes later, he returned. Mom was still in the same position.

He placed his hand on her shoulder and said, "Mrs. Frazzetto, you know you shouldn't be here. I am sorry, but I will have to ask you to leave."

Mom stared at him with unseeing eyes and said, "OK, I will leave in a few minutes." The nurse nodded his head. Mom was reluctant to leave me but she knew she had pushed the limit. Kissing my hand she said, "Mi-Mi, in your mind I want you to pray to St. Irene. She will grant us our miracle. Sleep well, and I love you."

Sleep never came. Sometime during the night the alarms on the respirator went off. There was something seriously wrong. I was having trouble breathing. I became frightened. The nurse checked the tubes that went from my mouth to the machine making sure everything was in place. After he did that, everything seemed to be back to normal. Minutes later, alarms went off again. Once again the nurse checked everything. Nothing was out of place. He was perplexed. He turned the alarm off, wondering what the problem was. This happened all throughout the night. The nurse could tell I was agitated. I tried to signal I was having trouble breathing. He tried to calm me down by saying "Michelle, try to sleep. Think of something that will soothe you, maybe the sound of rain-drops or perhaps the sound of a waterfall." I shook my head no. I tried to lift my hand to the respirator letting him know I was having difficulties. He stroked my arm and said "You need to relax. The machine keeps going off because you are upset and your breathing is labored."

Tears spilled down my face. In my mind I thought I was going to die. I willed myself to stay calm. I thought, maybe he was right. That wasn't the case at all. The machine kept going off. The other nurse in the room was getting frustrated with me. I heard him tell the nurse who was trying to help me say, "I wish she would die already. She has been here so long. It is time."

I was so scared. This man wasn't going to help me. He wanted me to die. I heard the nice nurse call someone on the phone. After a little while people began to come into my room. I heard a lot of different noises. They were changing out my machine as well as the tubes. I felt relieved something was being done. When everyone left, all was still and quiet. The nurse came back to my bed and said, "You are going to be OK. Try to rest." I closed my eyes and drifted away.

The following morning Mom came in bright and early. She immediately noticed something was different. She approached my bed and said, "Michelle, why do you have a new respirator machine?" She grabbed the magic slate, and placed it next to me. I began to write: "Tom saved my life."

Mom's eyes grew wide. Alarmed, she asked, "What do you mean?"

I began to write, "Can't breathe." As I was writing, the alarm on the respirator machine went off. I began to gasp for air. Mom ran out of the room looking for a nurse. One was already heading to my room. Mom followed her in to see what was happening. The nurse immediately went to the phone to call for a doctor. She asked Mom to leave the room. Minutes later a doctor came running down the hallway into my room. Once again my room was in chaos. Orders were being yelled. I heard the doctor ask the nurse to get Mom's consent for something. I wasn't sure what. The nurse went outside my door looking for Mom. She knew Mom wouldn't be far.

She said, "Mama, I need your permission to allow the doctor to give her a tracheotomy if it is needed."

Mom responded in despair, "No, I can't give you permission. Michelle told me she would rather die than have that put inside of her."

The doctor was listening to the discussion. He became irritated and lashed out at Mom, "I don't care if you don't sign the paper. I will do what I need to do. I am here to save lives, not end them." The door was shut abruptly in Mom's face. Mom stayed beside the door. She no longer could look through the window since they placed a piece of paper blocking the view. They had put it there from her last incident with the student. After a few minutes, she began to pace up and down the corridor with her rosary in her hands. It seemed interminable. She stared at my door, willing someone to come out of my room.

Finally the nurse did. She had a big smile on her face and said, "Mama, Michelle is breathing on her own. She is breathing on her own."

Mom released all her anxiety and began to cry. She repeated over and over "Thank you Lord Jesus, and thank you St. Irene for the miracle."

Mom still has the newsletter of St. Irene after twenty-eight years. She has it in a frame by her bedside.

...Be strong and courageous. Do not be terrified;
do not be discouraged. Only be strong and courageous!
...Do not be afraid; do not be discouraged...

JOSHUA 1:9,18; 8:1

CHAPTER NINE

The removal of my respirator was a pivotal point in my recovery. Mom was elated to hear I was breathing on my own. Eagerly waiting outside my room she paced up and down the hallway like a lioness in a cage. When they finally allowed Mom to see me she burst through the door. Tears of joy streamed down her face. She took my hand gently into hers, saying, "Michelle, you are strong. I knew you could do it. You will start getting better and better each day."

A nurse worked with me on breathing techniques and the use of my voice. Standing behind Mom with a big smile on her face she gained Mom's attention by saying, "Mama, Michelle can really use your help. She has breathing exercises to do four times a day." The nurse then showed Mom something like a funny-looking plastic mug with a mouthpiece attached to it. "Mama, this is a spirometer. This will help expand Michelle's lungs. She needs to put the mouthpiece in her mouth and take a deep breath. After she does that, she needs to blow into the tube as long as she can. There are numbers on the side. Michelle needs to reach the highest number possible." Mom listened intently. The nurse handed it over to Mom and said,

"Why don't you give it a try so you can see how it works?" Mom took the spirometer and tried it.

She looked up at the nurse and gave her word. "I will make sure Michelle does this four times a day, I promise."

The nurse smiled at her and said "You are a good mama. Michelle is very lucky to have you." She grabbed Mom and gave her a big hug.

Mom was true to her promise. We practiced the breathing technique four times a day. She also bought a little basket of silk flowers with a soft scent. The basket was no bigger than four inches long by three inches wide filled with little roses. In between my exercises we would practice with the little basket. Mom would place it under my nose and say, "Michelle, it is time to smell the roses. Take a deep breath in, and hold it, hold it, hold it." After twenty seconds she would say, "Okay, you can blow it out, out, out." We did this together every day, increasing a few seconds each day.

Every year Mom gives me a bouquet of roses for my birthday. I touch their delicate petals and take a deep breath indulging in the exquisite fragrance. Each time I do that it brings me back to the memory of when we practiced my breathing lessons together. It always puts a smile on my face, reminding me how far I have come since then.

Several days after removing my respirator the doctors gave the OK to have some of my bandages removed. They told Mom they would begin in the areas that I had suffered with second degree burns, exposing small parts of my body at a time. Mom was so excited. She held my hand and said "Michelle, guess what?" I could hear anticipation in her voice.

I responded in a hoarse voice, "What?"

Kissing my hand she said, "They are going to remove some

of your bandages today. Your skin is beginning to heal. I think they will first take off the ones on your legs." I gave her a faint smile. Excitement crept through my body. My expression quickly changed into a frown. Mom noticed and said, "What is wrong?"

I began to cry. "I'm so scared my legs will have scars all over them."

Mom reassured me, "That isn't going to happen. You have beautiful, perfect long legs. God will make sure they remain the way he created them." In the midst of my tears I giggled. I thought to myself: I love her so much. She is so hopeful and positive.

Later that afternoon two of my favorite nurses came in. They stood on each side of my bed. They were both very animated. The one who resembled me said, "Michelle, I am sure Mom told you we are going to take the bandages off your legs."

I nodded my head. The other nurse spoke with laughter in her voice, "We are waiting for your mom to get back from church. If we did this without her being here, we would be in big trouble with her." We all laughed together. On cue Mom walked into the room and we laughed even louder. Mom looked a little confused. She didn't know why we were laughing. It didn't matter. She welcomed the sound of happiness in my room.

The nurses spoke privately with Mom, informing her what they were going to do. Mom held her breath, overcome with emotion. One of the nurses came close to my bed and said, "Babygirl, we are going to sedate you while we do this. Close your eyes and go to sleep. We will wake you when it is over."

Before drifting away I heard Mom in the distance say, "I love you. Everything will be perfect."

I was slowly waking up. I could hear voices coming from far away. My mind was fuzzy. The voices were getting louder and louder. They were calling my name. I suddenly remembered my bandages had been removed. I tried to clear my head. I could feel Mom's lips all over my hand and fingers. Joy overcame me. In my mind I thought: They must have removed the bandages on my hands in order for me to feel Mom's gentle kisses. The fog in my head lifted immediately. In a hoarse voice I asked, "Ma, do I have any scars?" Mom's tears of joy fell on my hand as she said, "There are no scars, Mi-Mi. Your legs, arms, and hands are perfect."

The feeling of happiness was overwhelming. I reached up to wipe away the tears from her face. It had been so long since I was able to feel anything. I rested my hand on her face and said, "I love you Ma. Thank you for everything."

The two nurses were standing behind Mom. They too were overcome with joy. One of the nurses came closer to my bedside and began to explain to me why they removed most of my bandages. As I listened I realized I couldn't see the nurse clearly. A frown creased my forehead. The nurse noticed. "Michelle, what is wrong? Are you having any pain?"

I shook my head, "No, but why can't I see you well?"

The nurse gently rubbed my arm. "Michelle, you are still healing. You have come a long way Babygirl, but the road ahead is still long. Be happy with today's achievements." I nodded. Before the nurse left, she explained to Mom, "I will be back shortly with medicated skin lotion. We have to lather her body twice a day with it, morning and night. She only has a very thin layer of skin and we need to help prevent the skin from tearing apart."

Suddenly I felt exhausted. I closed my eyes feeling happy. Mom looked over at me and said, "You had a very long day.

Just rest. I am going to call everyone to give them the good news." I nodded, and darkness enveloped me.

That night I was asleep when David came. He sat at my bedside, taking my hand into his, gently thumb-wrestling with me. In my sleep, the gesture seemed so familiar. I awoke knowing he was there. I smiled at him, trying to focus on his face. I could barely see him. Again I thought: Why can't I see him clearly? Am I still deeply medicated?

David was thrilled when he got the news of my bandages being removed. Still playing with my hand he said, "Moo-Moo, I am so happy for you. You are getting better every day. Continue the good work and come home to me." I giggled when I heard him use my nickname. We talked about his recent trip to Cape Cod with his college friends. The trip had been planned before I got sick. David didn't want to go without me. Mom had insisted he go. He brought me a small gift, a white sweatshirt where the neckline and sleeves were cut off. The front of the sweatshirt had two beautiful blue eyes, a pink little nose, and lips with a few whiskers. Underneath the face was a beautiful rose and in the corner it said Cape Cod. He looked at me anxiously, hoping I would like it. I took it into my hands, indulging in the softness of the material. I looked at him smiling and said, "Thank you for thinking of me. I love it. I will wear it when I get home."

Before he left, he gently thumb-wrestled with me again and said, "I will see you tomorrow night. Remember, I will never leave you. I will always stay by your side. I am stuck on you the way peanut butter sticks to the roof of your mouth."

I giggled. My heart was filled with so much love for him. David made me very happy, and he gave me the strength to continue to fight the battle. I had no doubt he loved me. He stood by my side all this time regardless of my condition or what I looked like. Inwardly I thought how lucky I was to have him in my life. Every night when he left me he repeated the same words. "I will see you tomorrow night. Remember, I will never leave you. I will always stay by your side. I am stuck on you the way peanut butter sticks to the roof of your mouth." He did this until my very last day in the hospital.

The following day Mom entered my room with such exuberance. She had so much to tell me. A social worker had approached her about possibly staying in a room at the Ronald McDonald House. She didn't feel comfortable leaving me alone yet. She decided to talk to me about it. She sat beside me and began by saying, "Mi-Mi, a social worker came to see me this morning. They have a room at this house across from the hospital. They want me to stay there. They don't want me to sleep in the elevator room anymore."

Puzzled, I repeated after her, "Elevator room? Where is that? How long have you been sleeping there? What are you sleeping on?"

Mom hung her head. She seemed to regret telling me. She finally looked up at me and said, "The elevator room is a little area in front of the service elevator. I have been sleeping there for seven weeks on a small loveseat."

Tears filled my eyes. I was so hurt she sacrificed and suffered so much for me. I reached for her hand and said, "Ma, I am so sorry, I didn't know. Yes, I want you to go to the Ronald McDonald house. I want you to go and sleep on a bed." Tears spilled down my face. I felt so guilty.

Mom wiped my tears and said, "Mi-Mi, I didn't tell you this to make you feel bad. I wanted to be here. I couldn't leave you here alone." At that moment the blood pressure monitor began to beep. It caught Mom's attention. She realized the blood pressure cuff was still on my arm. She stood up, asking, "Michelle, how long has this been on you?"

I answered "All night and all morning."

Mom went wild. She left my room in an instant. Turning back to me she said, "I will be right back. I am going to get a nurse." A few minutes later Mom and the nurse came in. The nurse lifted my arm to remove the blood pressure cuff. Mom stood on the other side of the bed watching her. When the nurse unfastened it and removed it from my arm, the skin on my upper arm peeled off with it. Mom gasped in horror. I screamed in pain. The nurse immediately increased my medicine to sedate me. She then went to get silver sulfadiazine patches to place on the open wound, wrapping my arm in gauze. Mom just stood there and cried. When the nurse finished Mom looked the nurse squarely in the eye and said angrily, "What nurse was on duty last night? I am not here for one night and this is what happens to her?"

The nurse came around the bed to calm Mom down. She said cautiously, "Mama, I will report this to the head nurse. I am not at liberty to give her name. You need to speak to him."

Mom lashed out and said, "Michelle has been through so much. She doesn't need to suffer anymore. We just pulled her out of the grave." The nurse nodded her head in agreement.

When I finally awoke I realized my arm had been bandaged. I looked around for Mom. She sat quietly in the chair praying. I called out to her. She quickly came over to the bed. She took my hand and kissed it. I said, "Am I alright?"

Mom nodded her head and said "Yes. They had to put the silver sulfadiazine patches back on. When the skin heals again they will remove it."

I asked Mom, "Can you please raise the back of my bed a little so I can look out the window?"

Mom replied gently, "I will raise it just a little bit. I don't want the patches of silver sulfadiazine to fall off your upper chest." It was the one area in which I suffered third degree burns. It had been one of the last areas to heal because the patches continually fell off, ripping any skin that was there. In addition it wasn't a fleshy part of the body, making it difficult for the skin to grow back. The other area having trouble healing was the middle of my back. The slightest move I made or when the nurses had to change my sheets the patches would come off. It frustrated Mom how the patches constantly fell from my body. An idea occurred to her when she visited the fireman across the room. He had special elastic netting that held his patches in place in certain areas of his body, such as his legs, knees, arms, and so on. It was like a light bulb went off in her head. She came over to me and said, "Mi-Mi, I will be right back." She had this goofy look on her face. I knew she was up to something. After a beat she was back with a nurse, talking at the fireman's bedside.

I could hear the nurse tell Mom, "OK, I will bring you some. That sounds like a great idea if you can do it."

Mom came back to my bed with this huge smile on her face. She was excited. She sat down and said, "I am going to make you a vest out of mesh to hold the patches in place so your skin can heal and we can raise the bed a little more." I smiled at her and laughed. I knew Mom would be able to make it. She loved to sew. She was an amateur seamstress. The nurse came in with the roll of netting and other supplies. Mom sat there diligently working on her creation. I slept while she did that. I awoke to the sound of a small squeal and a clap of her hands. Cinderella's dress was finished.

Voilà! Mom's fashion creation was done. She brought it over to show me. She placed it into my hands so I could feel it. I held it closer to look at it. It seemed interesting but I really couldn't figure it out. Mom began to explain her invention, "Mi-Mi, I took the netting that is shaped like a tube and cut it open, making one large piece. I took two of those pieces, one for the front and one for the back. I threaded ribbon on the top by the shoulders, and along both sides from your underarm to your waist. I then cut around the neck to make a neckline, and around the arms to make it more comfortable for you." I was so proud of her I giggled. I knew she would come up with something.

I asked her, "How are you going to put it on me?"

She answered confidently, "We will untie the sides, place it over your head, and then tie the sides together." I was excited for her and for myself. I thought: If this works, my patches will stay in place and my skin will begin to heal faster.

I looked over at Mom, encouraging her, "Ma, go get the nurse and show her. I want to see what she thinks." Mom sprung out of her seat and off she went. A few minutes later they both came in. Mom enthusiastically described how she made the vest. The nurse picked it up, turned it around, and looked at it. A big smile lit her face.

She declared, "Mama, this is great. You did an incredible job. We can certainly use you here at the Burn Unit. You would be a big asset to us." Mom stood there proudly. Her face beamed with happiness. The nurse eagerly helped me try on my new vest. They slowly placed it over my head being careful not to touch the silver sulfadiazine patches on my back and chest. They tied the sides closed. They took a step back and looked at Mom's brilliant work. The nurse said, "Michelle, I think this is going to work. Your Mama is a genius. I am sure we will be making these vests for many years to come." She then hugged Mom and thanked her, "Mama, you have been a great help to all of us. We are going to miss you when Michelle goes home."

Each day brought new achievements and challenges. Finally, the booties on my feet were going to be removed. They still caused me a lot of pain. I was glad to be getting rid of them. Once again my anxiety level was high. No one knew how my feet had healed. I worried they would be deformed and I would possibly not be able to walk on them again. Mom and the nurse were in the room. Mom was very excited. She rubbed my hand in anticipation. She knew from the expression on my face I was nervous. She caressed my cheek and said, "Mi-Mi, I want you to smile. Everything will be OK."

I smiled at her nervously, uncertain of the outcome. The nurse was ready to remove the first one. My heart was pounding. I heard the sound of the strap being pulled away from the boot. The thumping of my heart grew faster and faster. In one swift moment the boot was taken off. My foot was free. It began to tingle. It was a feeling that now seemed so foreign. As I lay there trying to comprehend all that I was feeling, I briefly felt a soft tickle on the bottom of my foot. I looked wide-eyed at Mom. She stood at the end of the bed with a huge smile on her face. She winked at me and said, "I told you. A little bit of suffering, and your foot is perfect. You will now be able to wear your high heels."

Tears trickled down my face. The nurse said to both of us, "OK, I am ready to remove the other one. Are you two ready?"

Mom and I both nodded our heads. The second one was taken off. Once again Mom tickled the bottom of that foot. I laughed. I asked, "Is that one perfect too?"

Mom and the nurse answered in unison "Yes!" Mom came over to me and hugged me. Happiness filled my room.

Later that evening the nurse came in to lather my body with the lotion. While she waited for the pharmacy to send it up she monitored all my vital signs. There had been something I wanted to ask her, but I wasn't sure I should. The nurse sensed I had some kind of anxiety. Knowing something was on my mind, she asked, "Michelle is everything OK? Are you having any pain?"

I shook my head and said, "No, I am not having any pain, but I did want to ask you something."

Her expression grew serious. "What is wrong?"

Once again I shook my head and said, "No, nothing is wrong. I was just wondering why I don't have any fingernails and toenails. They feel really weird."

The nurse pulled a chair over closer to the bed. Taking my hand she said, "Michelle, we had to remove the skin from your hands. When we did that, your fingernails came off with it. As for your toenails, they came off while you had the booties on your feet."

I looked away from her, not understanding. Tears pricked the back of my eyes. Softly I said to her, "Will they grow back?"

Sadly she responded, "Honey, I really don't know. You will have to ask the doctors."

I was confused. I sharply turned my head to look at her. Alarmed, I said, "What about my hair? Will that grow back?"

Again she responded, "You really should ask the doctors those questions." Squeezing my hand gently she continued,

"Michelle, you have come a very long way. Please don't let little things like that bring you down. It is a miracle you are alive."

I no longer could hold my tears back. They spilled down my cheeks. The phone in the room rang. The nurse excused herself to answer it. She was silent for a moment, and then I heard her say, "I need that tonight. No! It can't wait till morning. If we don't put any on her, the skin will break open." After a few minutes she hung up abruptly. I knew something was wrong. She came over to me and said, "I will be right back."

A half hour later Mom came in. I asked, "Ma, have you seen the nurse? She was upset about something."

Mom nodded her head. "The pharmacy doesn't have any medicated skin lotion and it is critical they put it on you. Your skin is so thin and fragile. If they don't put a moisturizer on it, your skin will split and begin to bleed."

Right at that moment the nurse came flying into the room with a box in her hands. She had a big smile on her face. She said, "Mama, I am so glad you are still here. I am going to need your help. I found a box of samples of the lotion. I looked everywhere for it and found some in a closet." Excited, she said, "Mama, I need for you to cut the bottom of the tubes so it will come out quicker. And if you can Mama, it will be a great help if you can squeeze the tubes on Michelle's body and I will massage it in."

The assembly line began. Mom began to cut the tubes and squeeze them onto my body, and the nurse began to rub it all over. When they were done the nurse looked at me and Mom. "I'm glad I found those samples. This will hold you over until tomorrow. Thanks for your help Mama. We will have no setbacks when it comes to Michelle." With that being said, the three of us smiled at one another, feeling relieved.

It was the first week in September. My birthday was coming up. I couldn't believe how much time had passed. The last vivid memory I had was in July. My sense of time was all jumbled in my mind. Mom was now staying at the Ronald McDonald House. Her room at the house was very small, only six feet by nine feet, but it had a bed for her to sleep on. Dad would stay with her on the weekends. She had a nine o'clock curfew at the house. If she wasn't there before that time they would lock the doors. It upset her to leave me that early every night. Before she left she made sure she knew what nurse I had for the night. All the nurses had been wonderful to me except for the one who wished aloud I would die, and the other nurse who left the blood pressure cuff on my arm. We still weren't sure who that nurse was. I just figured it was a mistake on her part. I was terribly wrong.

One night she came in to do her rounds of the patients of the room. I realized it was her from the sound of her voice. She stood nearby beside another patient's bed. I was in terrible need of the bed pan. I called out to her and she ignored me. I waited a little while longer and tried to get her attention. Once again she ignored me. I began to panic. I had to relieve myself. I pressed the call button thinking that is what I had to do. I had been out of it for so many weeks I thought maybe there were rules to follow. She disregarded the bell too. I finally shouted, "Nurse, please can you give me the bedpan? I really have to go. If you don't, I'm afraid I might wet the bed!"

She stormed over to my bed, glaring at me, and in an icy tone she said, "If you wet your bed, I will leave you in those sheets all night long. You are not the only patient in this room. I am helping someone else." With that she walked away, leaving me forsaken and helpless.

In a last attempt, I yelled out, "Please, just hand it to me. I will put it underneath myself." It fell on deaf ears. I held on as long as I could. She went about her business with the other patients disregarding my needs. Ultimately I was forced to relieve myself wetting the bed. Tears of humiliation fell down my cheeks. All sense of dignity was gone. She was good on her word. She left me in wet sheets all night. Sometime during the night I awoke to someone taking my hands and tying my wrists to the bed rails. Sheer panic lanced through me. I realized it was the nurse. Terrified I said to her, "What are you doing? Why are you tying my wrists to the bed rail?"

Nastily she responded, "You are trying to pull your tubes and wires. So I have to restrain you from doing that." I was in disbelief. She was crazy. I wasn't trying to pull anything. I tried to withdraw my hand from her. She was much stronger; I didn't have a chance. For the second time that night, tears came. I didn't know why this nurse was treating me this way. I willed myself to fall asleep, praying for this night to end and the light of dawn to appear.

In the wee hours of the morning I heard voices in the hallway. The doctors were making their rounds. There were several of them. They would always go through my chart, discussing my progress and different treatments. Occasionally they would talk to me and ask me questions. On this morning I hoped they didn't ask me anything. I was extremely nervous; my hands were still tied and I didn't want them to see. Prior to falling asleep a thought had crossed my mind: The nurse had most likely been reprimanded for the blood pressure cuff, and now was retaliating against me. I wasn't about to tell the doctors what she had done the night before, putting myself in greater risk with the nurse, but one of the doctors noticed the discoloration of my hands. When he tried to lift my hand he realized it was tied at the wrist. He frowned and said, "Why are you tied up?" Alarm crept through me. I was speechless. I didn't know what to say. I looked around fearfully to see if the nurse was there. Behind the curtain I heard the nurse rustling. I remained silent. She said slyly, "Oh, I can explain. She tried to pull all her lines during the night so I had to restrain her."

I wanted to scream out. In my head I yelled: Liar! Liar! Liar! At that moment I realized she had forgotten she had left me tied up. She came around the curtain giving me a wicked look, challenging me to say something contrary to what she just said. I looked at her defiantly, not giving in to her but inwardly I felt defeated, not wanting to cross her. The doctor immediately gave her orders to remove them. She smiled sweetly at him and said, "I was just going to do that before you came in. I have to change her sheets. She wet them a little while ago. She wasn't able to hold her bladder. She couldn't wait for me to give her a bedpan." I wanted to jump out of my bed and strike her. She was humiliating me in front of all the doctors. I said nothing. I stayed calm. Inwardly I thought: I will tell Mom. She will handle it. I will never have this nurse abuse me ever again. The next three hours seemed like forever. Mom normally came in shortly after the changing of shifts. I waited anxiously.

Finally I could hear Mom's voice outside the door. She always came in with a smile. She opened the shades and came over to my bed. She noticed immediately something was wrong. She took my hand. Rubbing gently she said, "Mi-Mi, what is wrong? Did you have a bad night?" I began to cry. I was so afraid to say something to her. I didn't want to create any problems for myself. Mom grew impatient and demanded,

"Mi-Mi, what is wrong? Are you in pain? Did something happen to you?"

I composed myself and said, "Ma, the nurse last night wouldn't give me a bedpan and I wet the bed. She left me in wet sheets all night. During the night she tied my hands to the bed rails. The doctors noticed and she lied to them." Mom was outraged.

"Do you know who it was?"

I replied, "Yes, it is the same nurse who left the blood pressure cuff on me." Mom stood up ready to attack. I squeezed her hand, stopping her. I cautioned, "Ma, we have to be careful what we say. She may retaliate again and do other things to me." Mom nodded her head in agreement. Her whole body trembled with anger.

She patted my hand and said, "You don't have to worry about this. You worry about getting better and getting out of here. I will take care of it, I promise." That she did. I never again had that nurse on any of my shifts. Every night when Mom left she made sure I only had our favorite nurses. If there was a nurse not to her liking she made sure the nurse got switched. The head nurse of the night shift argued with Mom each time but ultimately relented, always making her happy. When Mom left my room for the night she put the chair beside my bed and put the bedpan on it. That way I could never be humiliated again.

It was my birthday. One of the Latino nurses was taking care of me that day. She was so excited for me. She entered the room humming a Spanish song. She came over to me and said, "Babygirl, I am going to make you more beautiful than what you are. It is your birthday, and everyone will be in to see you." I smiled at her. I loved her enthusiasm. She placed a few things on my bed. It looked like makeup and a colorful scarf.

I asked her, "What are you doing? What are those things on my bed?"

She laughed and said, "I am going to surprise you. Just wait and see." At that very moment Mom walked in with a brilliant smile. She saw the nurse apply something on my face and said, "What are you doing?"

The nurse laughed and said, "Mama, I am making Michelle beautiful for her birthday. I'm putting on some powder to tone down the redness in her face."

Mom became alarmed. "Is that OK to do?"

Still smiling the nurse responded, "Yes, Mama. I got the OK from the doctors." Mom relaxed, enjoying the moment. The nurse then picked up the colorful kerchief putting it over my bald head. She tied it to the side, just like the Spanish women wore it. She fussed with it until it was perfect. She stepped back to look at her work and said "There, you look gorgeous, my Babygirl." Mom clapped her hands with happiness. She said "Yes, Mi-Mi, you look beautiful. I can't wait for everyone to see you."

Each of my family members had only ten minutes with me. Sal and Jeanette were the first ones to come in. Sal had brought me a giant jelly donut that he made at the donut shop where we worked together. The donut was twelve inches in diameter. I laughed when I saw it. I still wasn't able to eat any food. I asked him to give it to the nurses so they could enjoy it.

Nick and Glenda came in next. They weren't able to bring the boys in to see me. I longed to see them both. They were surprised to see me all made up. They thought it was great the nurse did that for me.

Later my Uncle Giovanni came to see me. It was his first time up. He was in total disbelief when he saw me. I looked

149

nothing like myself. He handled his shock well and never let on to my change in appearance. As a gift he brought me a picture of Jesus. When he handed it to me he said, "My beautiful niece. I don't know why this had to happen to you. God will always be by your side to protect you." I was not allowed to keep the picture in the room. I was still in the Intensive Care Unit. Mom brought it to her little room at the Ronald McDonald house.

Teresa called from Italy during the day. The nurse brought the phone over to my bed so I could briefly talk to her. To top the day off David came in later that evening to spend a few hours with me, ten minutes at a time.

It turned out to be an awesome day, considering how bad the situation still was. My heart was filled with so much happiness. Days like this gave me the hope and strength to get better.

...if you could have done so, you would have torn out your eyes and given them to me.

GALATIANS 4:15

CHAPTER TEN

The doctors and nurses continued to express amazement with my progress. Although I had made many achievements I had much more to accomplish. The fireman with whom I shared the room had gone home. Another patient was still in the room with me. Patients came and left but I always stayed.

I was considered an old-timer. Only a few of us old-timers remained in the intensive care unit. Jon-Pierre was one, and another was a little baby across the hallway from my room. Baby Ramona was only ten months old. She had been burned by a firecracker. Her Mama put her in her crib to sleep on the Fourth of July. Baby Ramona's window was open. People were lighting fireworks. One went through her window landing in her crib. The sheets went up in flames, engulfing her. Ninety percent of her body was burned. She lost one of her ears and most of her fingers on both hands. Her face and body were severely disfigured.

Shortly after my birthday Baby Ramona celebrated her first birthday. Her parents brought in a beautiful dress for her to wear. They carried her up and down the hallway to show everyone. Mom was sitting with me when she heard activity outside my door. She went to see what it was all about. When she returned, she had visitors with her. It was Baby Ramona and her mom. They brought her over to my bed and introduced me to her. I rubbed her little arm and said, "Hello Baby Ramona. You must be the baby I hear crying across the way in the middle of the night."

Her mom said apologetically, "I'm sorry if she keeps you up at night."

I smiled and reassured, "Oh, no, Baby Ramona doesn't keep me up at night, the nurses do. She keeps me company after the nurses wake me up." We all laughed.

It was the first and last time I saw Baby Ramona. Shortly after her first birthday she died. On the night she passed, it was chaotic. Doctors and nurses were coming in and out of her room, barking unintelligible orders; nurses scrambling up and down the hallway. I had a gut feeling it wasn't good. I was seized with dread. When things finally settled down and all was quiet, it seemed eerie. I had a difficult time falling asleep that night not knowing if they had stabilized her or if she didn't make it. I listened for her cries, sounds that never came. When sleep finally fell upon me, I dreamt of Baby Ramona, and I knew she didn't make it. The following morning when Mom came in to see me, I could tell from her demeanor something was wrong. She did the usual. She opened the shades, brought a chair beside me, took my hand, and said "Good morning, Mi-Mi. How did you sleep?"

I looked at her and asked tentatively, "Is Baby Ramona gone?" Mom looked surprised.

Rubbing my hand she said, "Yes, she died last night. She was too young to survive her injuries. How did you know?" Tears fell down my face. I felt so angry inside.

I responded, "I heard a lot of commotion coming from her room. How fair is it, a little innocent baby has to die?"

Mom wiped my tears away and said, "Michelle, don't cry. Just remember her always." For a long time I thought I could still hear her cry in the middle of the night. Every Fourth of July I fondly remember Baby Ramona.

If I had any illusions in my head that my torture was over I was sadly mistaken. Physical therapy and occupational therapy had begun slowly but surely. They started working my legs and arms at a very slow pace. My whole body still hurt because of the trauma it went through. They had to be extremely careful with my skin since it was still very fragile. All therapy was done at my bed. I was in very bad shape. All of my muscles had atrophied from lying in bed for over two months. I couldn't believe how much my body had changed. I weighed no more than sixty-five pounds. I wasn't able to take a single step without collapsing to the ground. I couldn't hold a simple piece of silverware in my hand. Grasping a glass and lifting it to drink was impossible. A very long road lay ahead of me, made even more challenging because my eyesight continually failed me. Everything I did was more difficult. Since I was in a less sedated state it became clearer to me what I had gone through and what I was facing.

With each session of therapy I became angrier and angrier. Resentment started to filter throughout my body. I was emotionally not able to comprehend why something as tragic as this happened to me. Depression slowly settled in. Mom noticed my change in attitude and she didn't like it. One day after physical therapy she entered my room and found me crying. Mom always stayed out of my room while I had therapy. She couldn't handle listening to my cries of agony.

Her heart bled for me, for everything I was going through. If she could take all of my pain away, she would. She approached my bed and kissed my tear-stained face and said, "Mi-Mi, what is wrong? Why are you crying? Did they hurt you?" I was so angry at the world. It just wasn't fair what happened to me. I couldn't even look at her.

I stared straight ahead and said, "I wish I would have died! I hate what has become of me!" Mom took a sharp breath. It was as if someone had just put a stake in her heart. She was shocked I had said that. She hung her head as tears trickled down her face. All was quiet between us. I felt horrible inside. Guilt overwhelmed me. I was lashing out at the wrong person. I reached out to hold her hand and said, "Ma, I am so sorry. I just can't believe what has happened to me. I will never be the same again."

Mom wiped her tears away and said, "Michelle, you have come a long way. You will always be the same person. Nothing has happened to you on the inside. Your heart remains the same." We both began to cry in earnest.

Mom and I heard footsteps. Nick entered the room and inquired, "Why are the both of you crying?"

Mom responded, "Michelle is having a hard time with all that has happened to her, and she is becoming depressed."

Nick understood my frustrations. He tried to lift my spirits by saying, "Michelle, the worst is over. The Firebird is waiting for you to come home, to drive it again. So show this place what you are all about and get out of here." We laughed through our tears. Nick always managed to make me feel better. I tried to focus on his face. He was blurry. I blinked a few times to try to clear my vision and nothing changed. My eyes constantly burned. They were always terribly sore and getting worse every day. We had requested an ophthalmologist to come and check my eyes. I was anxious to find out what the problem was. As we were visiting with Nick the eye doctor came in. He introduced himself to all of us. He came over to me and had me do little tests. He looked at my eyes with a penlight. He then had me follow the light as he moved it. He put fingers in front of me to count them. I had some difficulties with that task. His fingers were so blurry I thought there were more fingers than what he put up. He turned to speak to Mom and Nick. The eye doctor said, "I am going to clean inside her eyes. I must remove the residue of mucous membrane that has sloughed off. I am not sure if the both of you want to be present for this."

Mom spoke up and said, "I am staying with Michelle. Doctor, you have no idea what I have witnessed the last few months." He nodded his head and looked at Nick. Nick nodded his agreement with Mom and affirmed he was staying too. The doctor opened some sterile swabs. He lowered my bottom lid and gently began to clean inside my eyes.

When he was getting ready to raise the upper lid he advised, "Michelle, this will be painful but I will clean your eyes as quickly as I can." I held my breath. My heart began to pound. I clenched my fingers into fists anticipating the pain. I felt something sharp swiftly go across my eyeball, up into the eye lid. I didn't flinch. I didn't move a muscle. I held my cry of agony until he was done. I thought I was going to pass out from the pain. The doctor touched my arm and said, "It is over. You did really well. You are an incredibly strong girl. I will see you upstairs in the ophthalmology department every couple of days to check your eyes."

I looked at Nick with tears in my eyes and said, "Nick, how do my eyes look? Do they look better?" Nick was horrified with what he just saw the doctor do. He was in utter shock with the appearance of my eyes. They looked like two red balls of fire. He couldn't see the sclera, iris or pupil. He felt sick to his stomach. He composed himself and reassured me, "Michelle, they are fine. You look beautiful." I smiled at him, feeling comforted by his answer.

The nurse came in to apply ointment inside my eyelids. She spoke to us both, "Mama and Michelle, it is critical that we put ointment in your eyes every hour. Hopefully this will help with the redness and soreness you are feeling, making them feel more comfortable." The first hour passed and the nurse wasn't back to put the ointment in. The nurses in the burn unit were always so busy. Burn patients always required so much attention. Mom was getting a little antsy. She allowed another half-hour to go by. Finally the nurse scurried in, putting sterile gloves on, apologizing to Mom and me. We didn't need any apologies. We certainly understood. Mom, always being sympathetic towards the good nurses, had an idea. As the nurse applied the ointment Mom said to her, "I know all you nurses are very busy, and an hour goes by very quickly. How about I give you a helping hand and put the ointment into Michelle's eyes?"

There were several reasons why Mom suggested she help. The first reason was the most important. She would make sure the ointment was being applied timely. The second reason was she would be able to stay with me the entire day. She was still limited to ten minutes every hour. The nurse smiled at her gratefully and said, "Mama, are you sure? You don't mind?"

Mom smiled back and said, "No, I don't mind at all."

The nurse hugged Mom and said, "You are the best. Thank you so much."

When Mom came in the following day, she found me sitting in a vinyl recliner chair. It was the first time she had seen me out of bed. One of the nurses was sitting beside me. The nurse had brought in a little radio and we were humming and singing to a song. Mom's heart swelled with joy. It was the best scene she had witnessed in a long time. With a broad smile she teased, "What are you two doing?"

The nurse smiled back. "Mama, we are listening to the radio and singing along. Michelle is young and she needs to get back into the groove of things." I laughed when I saw the look of shock on Mom's face. Mom shook her head, thinking we were both crazy.

The nurse stood up and said, "I have great news for you both. Today Babygirl, you can begin a liquid diet. If that goes well, you can start eating soft foods after that."

I couldn't believe my ears. It had been months since I could drink or taste anything. She proceeded by telling me what I would be able to eat: "You can have broth, juices, Jell-O, and... the highlight of the menu is ...plenty of 'high-calorie protein drinks.' Yuck!"

I giggled. All those things sounded heavenly to me. I was just so excited to taste something again. I had such a craving for water. I asked, "Can I have water? I have such a strong desire to drink some. I'm so thirsty for it."

She shook her head and said "No, you can't have water. Your potassium is very low so water isn't a good idea. You can have ice chips occasionally."

My liquid diet went well and now I had graduated to a soft food diet. That menu consisted of apple sauce, eggs, pudding, ice cream, milk, and everything that was on the liquid diet. Let's not forget the delicious "high-calorie protein drinks".

This menu was much more appetizing than the first one. Mom brought me chocolate milk every day. It was my special treat for the day. (Well, I thought it was a treat until I found out years later what she was putting in it. She would add an egg yolk so it would be more nutritious. Yuck!)

My progress was steady. The remaining areas of my skin finally healed. The bad news was those areas had scarred. I now had scars above my breast to my collar bone, on my upper right arm where the blood pressure cuff was left on, and in the middle of my back. They tried to fit me with a zippered garment applying pressure to help with the scarring. I couldn't wear it because the garment was too tight, hindering my breathing. I tried several times to wear it with no success. The darn thing felt like a straitjacket.

I was now allowed to take showers since all the bandages were removed. My first experience taking one wasn't pleasant. Mom wheeled me into a room down the hallway. The size of the room was six feet by eight feet and it was dimly lit. They allowed Mom to stay with me in case I needed help. Mom changed into hospital scrubs so she wouldn't wet her clothes. She tested the water to make sure the temperature was right. She wheeled me into the smaller confined area near the shower head. I reassured her I would be okay to wash myself. She turned away to set up her chair in the far corner of the room. With her back to me momentarily she couldn't see what was happening. I leaned my body and head forward beginning to wash my legs and feet. The water engulfed me. I panicked. My heart thumped rapidly. I struggled to move the wheelchair out of the way and I couldn't. The locks were on and I didn't have the strength in my hands to unlock them. I scooted forward in the chair trying to look over my shoulder for Mom. I couldn't see her. It only made the situation worse. The water was now directly spraying on my face. I thought I was there alone. I screamed out for Mom. When I did, I swallowed water, making me choke. I felt as if I was drowning. Shielding my face from the water, I began to cry. When she heard me yell she came quickly. Trying to calm me down she said, "Michelle, I'm here. What's wrong?"

"Water's hitting my face! I can't breathe!" Alarmed, she unlocked the chair and pulled the chair away. I felt relieved. I sat there and sobbed. I was ashamed. I couldn't even take a shower on my own.

Mom blamed herself for not remaining beside me. Clutching me in her arms she suggested, "We'll turn the wheelchair around so that the water hits your back first. We will soap you up and then face you towards the shower head to rinse you off. This way, the water won't constantly spray in your face. Mi-Mi, this is new to both of us. So, let's do it together and learn."

I looked at her with so much love. "But you will get soaked," I said.

She kissed my face. "I don't care if I get wet. All I care about is you." Each time I showered, she never left my side. She was good on her promise as usual.

My days were now a routine. Physical therapy and occupational therapy came after breakfast. I did my breathing exercises with Mom throughout the day. I took my showers after lunch so I was refreshed and clean for any visitors. Paulette had come to visit me once. She couldn't handle seeing me so sick; it emotionally affected her. Stacie would come to see me periodically, sometimes bringing my girlfriend Christine with her.

I desperately wanted to see my little nephews Nicholas and Michael. They weren't allowed to come into the Intensive Care

Unit. I figured out a way to see them. It was the last week in September. Michael's fourth birthday was three weeks away. My plan was to get the therapist to start walking me down the corridor to the doors that entered into the intensive care unit. It was a long hallway. I wasn't sure I could even do it. I wasn't walking at all at this point. I took a few steps here and there, but nothing that would be considered an achievement. I had my work cut out for me. I was so excited about my plan. I couldn't wait to surprise my family. I told all the nurses about my idea. They were thrilled. The only family member I shared it with was Mom. My determination paid off. I slowly made progress walking down the corridor. Every couple of days the therapist put an extra step into my session. I was really proud of myself. I couldn't wait to see the expressions on the faces of my loved ones.

One late afternoon Mom and Nick were visiting with me. Nick told me stories about what was going on in the outside world. I was a big Mets fan and so was he. He would tell me how well they were doing and how they were in the playoffs. Mom enjoyed these conversations. She was also a Mets fan. When I was a teenager I had taught her how baseball was played so she would let me watch the games on TV. We only had one television growing up, and we always had to watch what Mom and Dad wanted to see. Dad was never a problem. He just watched anything we were watching. Mom didn't understand the game. She would complain and say, "How can you watch that? It is so boring. All they are doing is standing with a bat, waiting to hit the ball, and the other players are waiting to catch it. How can that be exciting?" I would laugh every time she said that. I encouraged her to learn the game. And when she did she loved the sport just as much as I did.

Nick stayed a little longer than usual that afternoon. No one else was expected to visit. The nurses weren't so strict anymore with the time limit. Nick waited for Mom so he could walk her to church. When he visited in the evenings he stayed late so he could drive her to the Ronald McDonald House. Before leaving, Nick said, "Michelle, when you get out of here, I will take you to a Mets game."

I smiled at him. With excitement in my voice I said, "I am going to hold you to your promise!"

As Nick and Mom entered the elevator a doctor entered behind them. The doctor looked at Nick and said, "Hi, wasn't your sister the one who suffered with TEN (toxic epidermal necrolysis)? Did she make it? Is she still alive?"

Nick smiled at the doctor and said, "Yes, she is doing really well. She made it through TEN. She is walking and eating soft foods. If she continues doing well they are going to put her on another floor in a week or two."

The doctor's eyebrows shot in the air in surprise and said, "I'm glad. She is a miracle. You do know your sister will be blind, don't you?" Nick felt as if someone just kicked him in the stomach. Mom had been listening to the conversation. When she heard that she freaked out. Tears sprung immediately to her eyes. She wanted to scream out. Her body shook with rage. Nick clasped her hand trying to ease her pain.

When the elevator doors opened, Mom darted out of the elevator running for church. Once again she ran through the streets into traffic not caring for her own life. Nick ran after her trying to stop her. He yelled, "Ma, please stop! You are going to get yourself killed!"

Mom shouted back, "I don't care. I want to die!" She continued to dart in and out of traffic. She reached the church breathless.

Nick was right behind her. Mom tried the church doors and they were locked. She slumped to the ground, sobbing.

Nick went over to her, holding her close, and said calmly, "Ma, come sit on the steps with me." He held her in his arms, advising, "Ma, don't listen to the doctors. They don't know if Michelle is going to be blind." Mom continued to cry in Nick's arms. He tried to comfort her by telling her, "Michelle still can see. I know her vision is blurry right now. Maybe she won't be able to see perfectly but she won't be blind. Please don't worry."

Mom looked at him with her tear-stained face and asked, "How am I going to tell her?"

Nick wiped a tear and suggested, "Don't say anything to her. The doctors don't know everything Ma."

Mom nodded her head in agreement. She stood up. "I have to go back and see Michelle. I need to be near her."

Nick helped her down the steps, and walked her back to the hospital reaffirming, "Remember, not a word to Michelle."

When Mom entered my room I was surprised she had returned so quickly. She came over to my bed and kissed my cheek. I sensed something was wrong. I could tell she had been crying. I asked her, "Ma, what is wrong? You've been crying. Did Nick say something to you?"

She shook her head and said, "No. Nick was talking about the boys and I miss them. That is all." My heart went out to her. She had been away from home for a long time.

I took her hand reassuring her, "Ma, if you want to go home for one night, it's OK. I'm feeling better now."

Mom shook her head again and indicated, "No, I will go home when you go home. I will be OK." Mom sat there with a heavy heart. She stared into my eyes. Eyes that no longer looked normal. Her heart was broken for me and herself.

The following day Mom added another ritual to her routine. After she opened the shades, she came over to the bed and began, "Good morning Mi-Mi, how was your night?" I would give her my usual answer unless something happened during the night. She would continue by saying, "Can you see the color of my dress?"

I would look over at her and respond, "It is pink, with white stripes." Or whatever color dress she had on that day. Mom would nod her head with satisfaction.

She would then squeeze my hand and say, "That is right. Good job." I always gave her a peculiar look when she did that. I wasn't sure why she did this every morning.

Mom's anxiety grew each passing day after she heard what the doctor said in the elevator. She just expected to come in one morning and I would be blind. She expressed her concern to one of the nurses. In order to ease her mind they made an appointment for her and Dad to see the chief ophthalmologist who was treating me so they could hear his explanation about what was happening with my eyes.

Mom and Dad were nervous as they sat in the eye doctor's office. The doctor sat behind his desk, smiled, and introduced himself. He began by saying, "I understand you both have questions and concerns about Michelle's eyes." Mom and Dad both nodded. He continued, "The surface of Michelle's eyes burned just like her body did. It damaged the entire surface as well as her cornea, and that is why she doesn't see that well." Mom held her breath. She took Dad's hand in hers and continued to listen. The doctor proceeded, "I am not sure after all of this is done what the condition of her vision will be. We are doing our best to maintain what she has but nothing is guaranteed."

Tears pricked the back of Mom's eyes. She sat on the edge of the chair and said, "Doctor, will she be blind? Please, you have to tell me."

The doctor's expression was solemn. He responded, "Mrs. Frazzetto, I can't tell you what is going to happen because I really don't know. All I can say is Michelle will never have perfect vision ever again." Tears trickled down Mom's face. She was determined not to give up.

Uneducated in the medical world, Mom asked "Can my husband and I give one eye each to Michelle, so she can see?" The doctor looked at Mom and Dad both with admiration.

He replied compassionately, "I'm sorry Mrs. Frazzetto. That can't be done. Eye transplants are not possible. It just doesn't exist in the medical field." Mom began to cry in earnest. Dad tried to comfort her. The doctor looked at them sadly, recommending, "Mrs. Frazzetto, let's work on getting Michelle better and stronger. We will address her eyes when she is healthier and strong. There is a possibility of a cornea transplant, but we have to wait."

Mom and Dad left the office feeling defeated. They both sat on a bench in the hallway, holding each other, crying, consoling one another's hearts. They both knew at that moment my world of color and beauty as I saw it would never be the same.

My heart pounds; my strength fails me;
even the light has gone from my eyes.

PSALM 38:10

CHAPTER ELEVEN

Finally, the day arrived in which I would walk down the corridor to greet my family. My room buzzed with excitement throughout the day. I had worked so hard for this moment. My family didn't know what I was up to, except for Mom. All my nurses were going to help me achieve my goal in surprising them. I was still extremely weak. I had not reached the end of the hallway with my physical therapist during our sessions but I was determined to do it on this day. The nurses would accompany me on this walk. I would have a nurse on either side of me helping with the intravenous pole and there would be one nurse behind me and another nurse with a wheelchair in case I couldn't make it.

My family was waiting on the other side of the doors of the intensive care unit: Nick, Glenda, Sal, Jeannette, Mom, and of course my two little nephews Nicholas and Michael, who I wanted to see over anyone else, and the ones I most wanted to do this for. They were waiting with anticipation and excitement.

I sat on the edge of my bed listening for the nurses. So many different thoughts and emotions went through my mind. I was nervous, excited, frightened. My heart thumped fiercely in my chest. I was afraid I would not be able to walk the entire corridor. I didn't want to fail. I thought about calling it all off. Inwardly I knew if I did that I would never forgive myself for giving up and never taking on the challenge. For a brief moment I wondered what would it feel like to reach the doors. If I accomplished that, I would know I could go further someday where I could pick up the pieces of my shattered life and start putting it back together again. The nurse entered my room, interrupting my thoughts. With a smile on her face she said, "OK Babygirl, we are ready for you." My heart skipped a beat. Two nurses helped me to my feet. Holding me by each arm they both said, "Are you ready?" I panicked. I stood there paralyzed in place. One nurse said, "What is wrong?" Tears pricked the back of my eyes.

I explained, "I will feel like a failure if I don't make it all the way to the doors." The nurse rubbed my arm reassuringly and said, "You have worked very hard for this moment. If you don't reach the doors your family will be proud of you no matter what. Remember, at any point if you need to stop, just squeeze our hand. You can stop, rest, and continue."

I took a deep breath in and said, "OK, let's do it." Very slowly, each step I took was one step closer to my goal of reaching the doors and seeing my loving family.

As we continued the journey the nurses informed me of my specific location. I stopped several times to rest. There were other nurses, aides, doctors, patients, and their relatives cheering me on as I made my way. It empowered me to continue. My breathing was labored. My body bent with fatigue. All of me ached. My eyesight only allowed me to see somewhat clearly a few feet in front of me. Because I couldn't see in the distance, it caused me more anxiety to not know how close I was to my destination.

My family members took turns looking through the little windows on the doors, hoping to see me. They finally saw the first glimpse of me. Little Nicholas shouted, "She is coming. Aunt Mi-Mi is coming!"

They all prepared themselves for my arrival. The boys were so excited to be able to finally see me. Nicholas was five, and Michael was celebrating his fourth birthday.

As they watched each step they were flooded with emotions. Sal began to sob, saying to Nick, "She looks like she is coming back from the war." Tears fell down Nick's face. Glenda turned her tear-stained face away; she couldn't bear to see the agony on my face. Mom stood proudly as tears pooled in her eyes.

I was struggling. I thought I was going to collapse. My chest constricted with pain from breathing so heavily. I was about to squeeze the nurse's hand to let her know I couldn't continue when these magic words were uttered, "You have made it, Babygirl. We are going to open the doors so you can see everyone."

I stood there feeling exhilarated, anxious, exhausted. I heard all their voices at once. Words of praise filled my ears. They showered me with hugs and kisses. I began to cry. I'd made this effort for all of them. I wanted to give something back and thank them for the encouragement they had given me the last few months. The nurses sat me down on the wheelchair sensing my exhaustion. I was eager to hold my little nephews in my arms. I called to them, "Nicholas, Michael, come to Aunt Mi-Mi."

Michael began to cry. Between his sobs he said, "That isn't Aunt Mi-Mi! She doesn't look like Aunt Mi-Mi. I want my Aunt Mi-Mi!"

Nicholas held his little brother and said, "Mike, that is Aunt Mi-Mi. She is just sick. She has a boo-boo. When she gets better she will look like Aunt Mi-Mi." My heart tore in two. The emotional pain was unbearable. Michael's words were like a knife in my heart. Tears fell down my face like two waterfalls. I didn't understand. I had no idea what I looked like. Was I that horrific? I was emotionally bleeding inside. I wanted to escape. I didn't want to cause the boys any pain by seeing me this way. I'd wanted this moment to be a joyful one. I indicated to the nurse I wanted to go. I couldn't handle the hurt. At that very moment I felt Nicholas's little hand on my leg. He said, "Me and Michael want to give you a hug Aunt Mi-Mi. Is that OK?" My heart soared with such happiness, I took the both of them in my arms, holding them tight, never wanting to let them go.

The nurses brought me back to my room. I waited patiently for Mom. I had so many questions to ask her. Michael's outburst had bothered me. Mom came in. She could tell I was upset. She pulled a chair over to my bedside and said "I am so proud of you. Everyone is. I know it took a lot of strength and courage to do what you did today, and I love you for it." I no longer felt proud. I was ashamed.

I looked at Mom and said, "What do I look like? Why was Michael so afraid of me?" Mom took my hand and kissed it.

She explained gently, "Michelle, you have no hair, and your face is swollen and red from the medicines. Michael is accustomed to seeing you with your long blonde hair. He is a little boy and doesn't understand. Nicholas was okay with you." Tears trickled down my face.

I said, "I want to see myself. Bring me to a mirror."

Mom looked at me sadly. With compassion she said, "They don't have mirrors in this unit, Mi-Mi. When you get home you can look in a mirror all you want and you can see how beautiful you still are." Mom always managed to lift my spirits. Inwardly I thought maybe it wouldn't be a good idea to see myself in this condition. If I didn't recognize the person looking back at me it might spiral me into a deep depression. The thought scared me. A shudder ran through my body. I dismissed the idea immediately. The subject was closed and forgotten for the time being.

I had jumped another hurdle. They were going to move me to another room on a different floor. I would be leaving the burn unit of intensive care. It was the second week in October. I was progressing quickly. Just a few weeks before, the doctors and nurses were teasing me about staying long enough to play Mrs. Claus for Christmas. I had told them cheerfully I wouldn't be in the hospital to fulfill that role so they needed to find another candidate for it.

Privately my emotions were all over the place. I felt such trepidation leaving the one place I had considered home the last few months. It had become my safe haven. The knowledge I was leaving caused me severe anxiety inside. On the other hand I was thrilled and excited. Finally I was one step closer to going home. Although that thought made me happy, it also frightened me immensely. I imagined being part of society again and it made me scared and nauseous. I was so confused in my head and heart. How could I ever walk the sidewalks of New York City? I could barely walk down a hallway. I couldn't even see correctly anymore. I realized I was no longer the girl from a few months back. How could I resume my relationship with David? Would he have the patience to help me get back on my feet? Depression seized my soul. I just wanted to curl up in a ball and withdraw from everyone and everything. Mom noticed my complete despair.

The doctors were waiting for a room in order to transfer me downstairs. Inwardly I hoped it wouldn't happen. In the meantime I stopped trying so hard with physical therapy and occupational therapy, taking my progress a few steps back. I was struggling inside. My soul was in turmoil. Anger penetrated my being. I couldn't deal with all these different feelings. I wanted to scream out for help.

Mom was worried. She shared her concerns with Nick. One night when he came to visit he decided to try his tough-love theory on me. It didn't go well. Nick stood at the end of my bed. He was getting ready to leave, but before he did he said, "Mi, it is time you get your butt moving and get out of here. You need to start making more of an effort. You can't be lying around all of the time. I don't know how much longer Glenda and I and the boys can continue to come up. If you have decided to give up on yourself I just won't come to see you anymore."

Outrage sliced through me. What nerve he had! Did he think this was a freaking picnic? My eyes blazed into his. I shouted at him, "I am trying my best! Do me a favor, get the heck out of my room and don't come back!" Mom stood up in shock. She couldn't believe the ugly exchange between Nick and me. Nick turned away.

As he made his way out he said, "Okay, I will leave. Remember, I love you and I will see you when you come home." When he left I began to cry. Nick was the only constant in my life besides Mom, and David. Didn't anyone understand what I was going through?

I no longer shared my feelings with Mom. I withdrew. I decided to live in this hell all by myself. Mom was determined to have a talk with me to see what was really going on. She wasn't happy with the change of attitude I displayed. One afternoon she came in with my chocolate milk. She turned down the television and said, "Once you go downstairs you will be on a regular diet. The doctors said you need to consume four thousand calories a day." My eyes opened wide in surprise.

I answered, "How am I going to eat all those calories? I hate hospital food."

Mom laughed and said, "I know you do. Do you think I forgot what a fussy eater you are?"

"So, how am I going to be able to do that? I don't think I can drink anymore 'high-calorie protein drinks' than I am right now."

Mom took my hand and said tenderly, "I thought I could go home and make you all of your favorite meals." My heart lurched in my throat. Tears stung my eyes.

In a panic I said, "You mean you are not going to stay at the Ronald McDonald house anymore? You are leaving me?"

Squeezing my hand, she said, "Does that frighten you? Mi-Mi, I have noticed in the past week you haven't been the same. You have lost all your ambition to get better and get out of here." Why was she so wise and perceptive? I hung my head. A teardrop welled up. I felt so ashamed of myself for being insecure. Mom came over to me and hugged me. She sensed there was something else bothering me. The tears now spilled down my face. She gently searched, "Is that the only problem?" I shook my head no. She wiped my cheeks and offered, "Talk to me. Maybe I can help."

In between my sobs I said, "I am so afraid. All I have known the last few months is this room and the hospital staff. They have become my family and this place has become my second home." Mom suddenly saw my dilemma and her heart bled for me. Until that moment she had been confused with my reaction. She had just assumed I would be happy to leave the hospital and go home.

Mom sat on my bed and said, "Michelle, I know you are scared but you can't stay here forever. At some point you need to come home. What part of coming home makes you nervous?"

Punching my bed, I said "All of it. I am afraid I will have trouble breathing, and there isn't any equipment to help me. Walking up the stairs to my room!?—I can barely walk down the hallway. And David, what kind of girlfriend can I be to him as sick as I am? I am so afraid he is going to leave me. Right now he is *obligated* to come visit."

Mom took my hands and said, "I have solutions for everything. They won't let you go home without the proper equipment. I am sure they will have an oxygen tank sent to the house. You can sleep in Nonno's and Nonna's old bedroom on the first floor. They went to live with your Aunt. As for David I am sure he isn't going to leave you. He has been so dedicated, coming here every night and on the weekends while you were in the coma. He didn't have to do that. He would have left you already." Once again Mom had all the answers.

Feeling slightly better, I hugged her and said, "Mom, I love you. Thank you for always being here for me." After several days my room downstairs was finally ready for me to transfer. My excitement had grown after my talk with Mom.

David and I also had a talk one night when he visited. I was prepared to put my heart on a platter. I knew I had to do this. Although I didn't know what the outcome would be I had to take a chance with him. He looked so good in a business suit. I missed the days when we worked together and the days we went to lunch when I worked at Solomon Brothers. We looked great as a couple. I wondered if it would ever be that way again. David sat beside my bed, took my hand, and gently thumb-wrestled with me. I giggled. I loved this man so much I didn't want to lose him. I didn't want us to change. We talked about his day and all the drama in the office. Jill's name was never mentioned all the times he came to see me. She was probably disappointed I had survived. I am sure she still wanted to put her claws into my man. I laughed at the thought. I was feeling nervous. My heart thumped rapidly. I didn't know how I would bring up the topic of him and me, and our future together. David sensed something was not right. He asked me, "Is everything OK Moo-Moo? You must be very excited to be going to a regular room downstairs."

I shrugged my shoulders and said, "I am, in a way, but I also have a lot of hesitations." He looked confused.

He stated, "I don't understand. I thought you would be happy to get out of here and home." I looked down, not being able to meet his beautiful blue eyes. Once again he said, "What is wrong?"

I felt sick. I mustered all my courage and blurted, "I am so afraid once I go home you will leave me and I won't see you anymore."

Gently rubbing his thumb over my knuckles, squeezing my hand as reassurance, he said, "For the last several months I have been telling you the same thing over and over again whether you could hear me or not. I will tell you again tonight. I will always be here for you. I will never leave you. I am stuck on you just like peanut butter sticks to the roof of your mouth." My heart soared with love and happiness. Tears of emotion filled my eyes. He continued, "Things will be a little different in the beginning until you start feeling better, but I promise to come see you on the weekends. If you feel well enough to go for a drive or anything else we can do it." Those words were the only reassurance I needed. It was full speed ahead for me.

All my nurses reflected my renewed enthusiasm. They were happy to see me move on but they would miss me and Mom terribly. I promised once I was discharged I would come back and say goodbye to all of them. My bed in the new room was by a window. They knew I enjoyed the sunlight on my face. They tried to keep the room similar to the one I was in because of my eyesight. I had a beautiful black woman across from me. When I say beautiful, I mean she was beautiful on the inside. I didn't know what she looked like since all I could see was her silhouette. She made me laugh all of the time with her stories. We kept each other company during the day. I wasn't sure why she was in the hospital. She never said. One day they brought her down for a test. When she came back I asked her, "What did they do for you today?"

She responded in her sweet song voice, "They took me down for a chest x-ray. I'm not sure why they did that. There is nothing wrong with my chest. I'm having problems with my toe." She began to laugh. Her laughter was so infectious I began to laugh with her.

Mom went home every day to cook for me. She was my own personal chef. She would wake up at four o'clock in the morning to prepare my breakfast, lunch, and dinner. My breakfasts consisted of omelets, french toast, pancakes. For my lunches Mom would make my favorite sandwiches with prosciutto, capicola, mortadella, or anything else I desired. Dinners were always my special meals. She made me steak pizzaiola, veal cutlets, baked ziti, manicottis etc. She also made sure she brought me plenty of cupcakes, snack food, and juices. Mom would walk to the corner to get the bus. The bus would drop her off at the ferry, and when she got off the ferry she would take another bus to the hospital. She would arrive at my room at eight thirty in the morning. Passengers would make comments about the wonderful aroma of her food. Mom always managed to make acquaintances wherever she went.

After several days of this routine I began to feel extremely guilty. I felt as if I was an incredible burden to her. I expressed this to Mom one day as we sat together eating ice cream. I looked over at her and said, "Ma, you don't have to wake up so early every morning to prepare my food. I am feeling really badly about it. I can eat cereal and the cakes you bring me for breakfast, and for lunch and dinner you can get something from the nearby restaurants." I thought Mom was going to have an epileptic fit. I really did it this time. She looked like a cobra ready to strike.

She sat up in her chair and pulled back her shoulders and said, "I don't want you to feel badly about anything! I want to do this. I will not allow you to eat that garbage food. Is that clear?" I winced.

The black lady across from me with laughter in her voice exclaimed, "Loud and clear, Mama." We all laughed.

Mom continued with her ritual. Each morning I knew by her footsteps when she was approaching my room. When she was at the threshold I could smell the food. I would say to my friend across the room, "My Mom is here."

She would respond teasingly, "How do you know that? I don't see your Mom."

I would answer back, "I guess your eyesight is worse than mine," and, "You better have them take an x-ray of your nose because that isn't working either. Besides, if she was standing right there you wouldn't tell me anyways." Laughter would erupt in our room.

I continued with my physical therapy. It was becoming more and more challenging each day. I was no longer just trying to learn how to walk or how to hold my silverware properly again. I was learning how to do all these things as a visually-impaired person. It was a thousand times more difficult. In one of my sessions my physical therapist wanted me to walk from my bed to the door by myself. I gingerly took each step hoping I was walking straight. I had a tendency to lean to my left or right. I was concentrating on counting my steps to the door when suddenly I smacked my face into the wall. I screamed in pain thinking: Why didn't she help me? I was so angry I punched the wall with all I had. I wanted to grab the physical therapist by her hair. I yelled for her, and said "Where are you? Weren't you looking at me?"

Very calmly she responded, "I am here. Yes, I was watching you. You geared to the right and that is why you slammed into the wall. You have to learn to put your hands in front of you while you walk so it doesn't happen again."

I wanted to "strangle" her. I snapped at her, "You have no idea the hell I have been through the last few months. I don't need this humiliation from you. You could have warned me I was going in the wrong direction and corrected me. Or you could have simply reminded me to put my hands in front of me. This is all freaking new to me!" I wanted to slump to the ground and cry. Instead I took control of my anger and emotions, looked for the light coming from the window, and made my way back towards the bed by myself. I certainly wouldn't ask her for any help. As I walked away, I turned back over my shoulder and announced, "What just happened was a liability! This will be our last session together; I will make sure of it!" That was the last time I had physical therapy with her. Another therapist was assigned to me the following day.

One week later the ultimate good news was given to Mom. If my progress continued I would be leaving the hospital in another week. Mom was ecstatic. To me the news seemed unbelievable. I couldn't wrap my mind around it. The month of October had gone by so quickly. My projected date was October 28th. Again, all those insecurities came flooding back. I had just been transferred to my new room and was still trying to get acclimated to my new surroundings. Once I left the hospital I would no longer have its protection. My comfort zone would be abolished. But I also wondered how it would be outside of these walls. How it would feel to take in a breath of fresh air? ...To hear a bird chirp? ...To feel the sun directly on my face and not through a window pane? I had been a prisoner of concrete walls all these months. I would be free.

I was in awe of all these new feelings. Nervous anticipation quietly crept over me. I began to plan on what I was going to wear my first day home. I had lost so much weight. I wasn't sure if anything fit me anymore. Maybe I could have Mom bring me my favorite jeans with a belt and one of my comfy sweaters. (I certainly couldn't wear my heels—I *really* would lose my balance and fall flat on my face; never mind slamming against the wall!) I laughed at the thought. That would mean I would have to wear sneakers. (Boring!)

Mom had returned from church. The Mets game was going to be on TV. We would watch it together. The Mets had made it to the World Series. We were so excited. During the commercials Mom and I talked about what clothes to bring when I was discharged. Mom agreed that not all my clothes would fit. She promised to bring several different outfits just in case. The time had come for Mom to leave. It was eight o'clock at night and she had a long, two-hour trip home. She would miss the end of the game. If the Mets won, they would be the World Series Champions. I wished she could stay but I knew she was tired. One more week and her extreme sacrificing would be over. I couldn't wait to go home as the guilt overwhelmed me each day watching her give up her life for me. Mom came over to the bed and kissed me. With a wry smile on her face, she asked, "Are you going to sleep? Do you want me to turn off the television for you?"

I smiled back at her and said, "No, and no. I am staying up until it is over. I want to see if they win."

Mom laughed, "You know, a few innings can take hours. You don't want to disturb your roommate."

I looked at her menacingly and said, "I will lower the volume. Besides, I wouldn't be able to sleep not knowing if they won or not." (The Mets did win the World Series that year.)

It was D-day, "D" for discharge. I had butterflies in my stomach. Dad waited for us downstairs. I had not seen him in months. Mom brought my jeans and sweater as I asked. They didn't fit, not that they were too big; they were too small around my waist. I was swollen from the steroids. I was so upset. Thank God for Mom's good thinking. She'd brought me my designer sweat-suit that David had given me for Christmas.

During the last week David and I had begun a daily count-down. I couldn't wait to be with him outside this hospital. We made so many plans together. Our future promised to be strong. I would continue the hard work of rebuilding my life. This would be not only for me and my family, but for a life with David. I wanted him to be proud of me. I wanted to stand by his side and shine just like I did several months back. I had a lot of work ahead of me but I wasn't going to back down and give up in defeat.

I sat in the wheelchair waiting for the OK to leave. Mom and I wanted to go upstairs to the burn unit to say goodbye to everyone. I wondered if they even knew I was leaving. The last several weeks were like a whirlwind. Everything happened so quickly. The nurse came in with my final papers to sign. Mom eagerly signed them. Mom took the handles of the wheelchair and said, "Mi-Mi, are you ready to go upstairs?" I nodded my head yes.

We made our way through the doors of intensive care to the burn unit. Most of my nurses were on duty. When they saw me they cheered. They surrounded me, giving me hugs and kisses. Some had tears of joy in their eyes. Others had no control of the tears rolling down their cheeks. I thanked all of them for their amazing help, their compassion, and their infinite love not only for me but for my Mom.

My heart was heavy. I had grown to love all of these people. They were now part of my family. One of my favorite nurses asked Mom for her permission to have a girl-to-girl talk with me. This was the nurse who had introduced me to music again, the one who sat there and sang with me, and showed so much care and love. As she wheeled me down the never-ending hallway she said, "Okay, Babygirl, do not allow your Mom to pick out your clothes. Don't let her make you wear long black skirts with black shirts like the typical Italian woman. Make sure no chin hair grows out of your face. If it does, you pluck it. Make sure to always shave your legs and underarms." I was laughing and crying at the same time.

I vowed, "I promise never to let that happen."

She hugged me tight and whispered in my ear, "I love you, and I will miss you. I am so happy you survived. The road is going to be very long, Babygirl, but I know you can make it." I held on to her, never wanting to let her go.

When she pulled away from me she said, "One last thing. The next time you come visit I want to see you walk through those doors in your high heels." I laughed. I wondered how long it would take for me to do that.

As Mom and I departed, shouts of good wishes came our way. When we reached the infamous doors of intensive care, Mom turned me around in my wheelchair so we could face everyone. For the last time Mom looked at the familiar surroundings. Life-changing events had happened here. We both had so many good and bad memories. Parts of our hearts and souls remained behind. Tears spilled down our faces as we waved goodbye to everyone.

As Mom and I made our way towards the front doors of the hospital the realization about what was really happening struck me hard. Fear suddenly gripped me. My heart began to thump fiercely in my chest. A loud roar rang in my ears. I felt lightheaded. I thought I was going to pass out. I tried to take control of my fear. Before we reached the doors I shouted back at Mom, "Ma, please stop! Wait! Ma! Stop the darn wheelchair!" Mom continued down the hall, disregarding my pleas. Did she not hear me with all the noise around us? Or did I not say it aloud? I flipped up the footrests of the wheelchair and placed my feet on the floor. Mom stopped abruptly. In a panic she said, "What is wrong? What happened?" I covered my face with my hands trying to control the rhythm of my breathing. Mom came around the wheelchair and knelt in front of me.

Taking my hands away from my face, she asked, "Mi-Mi, what is wrong?" She searched my expression for an answer.

I was pale and stricken. I looked into her beautiful brown eyes and confessed, "I'm afraid. Once I go through the front doors, I don't know if I can handle what waits for me out there."

Mom hugged me tight. Understanding my fears and wiping my tears she said, "Michelle, I promise never to let anything happen to you. I will always be by your side."

I nodded, instinctively knowing that to be true. She put the footrests back into place and stayed by my side. She promised, "I won't move until you are ready. We will do this slowly, one wheel at a time." I laughed at her silly phrase.

I sat there for a few minutes regrouping, saying goodbye to this place in my thoughts. I could feel the cool breeze on my face as people came and went through the front doors. It was tantalizing. Dad was waiting for me on the opposite side. I desperately wanted to see him. I wanted to smell the familiar scent of cigarette smoke on him. Normally it would bother me but now I welcomed it. Inhaling deeply, I looked over my shoulder to Mom and said, "OK, I am ready."

A rush of cold air hit me as we went through the doors. I had to catch my breath for a minute. All that cool air at once was a shock to my lungs. I noticed the air wasn't totally fresh and clean. But it was the best Manhattan could offer. Mom stopped and said, "Are you OK?" I was awestruck. There were so many sounds that seemed foreign to me now: the roar of traffic, car horns, sirens, voices yelling for taxis, and crowds of people everywhere. My heart quickened. I nodded to Mom yes. But I was speechless.

She went a little further into the sunlight. I had to shield my eyes from it. It was a glorious October afternoon. The air was crisp and the sun was bright. The sun felt different on my face. It was much more intense than through a window. I sat there thinking: I am free from the concrete walls. It is time to put my life back together again. Dad's voice interrupted my thoughts. I could hear him shouting Mom's name above all the noise. Mom pushed my wheelchair towards him. Dad ran to me hugging me tight. Tears fell from his face. I noticed he didn't smell like smoke. (Mom had warned him not to smoke because of my lung condition.) Kissing each cheek I said to him, "Papa, I missed you. How have you been?"

Caressing my face he said, "Forget me. How are you? You look so much better. I missed you too." Once again he hugged me tight. Holding me by my arm Dad helped me to my feet and into the car. When he shut the car door I looked outside the car window trying to see the hospital for the last time. With anxiety I realized I was leaving the place that had saved my life. This was the place that had been my home for the last three months. All I could see was the outline and the color of the building.

My heart was filled with mixed emotions. I was excited to be going home yet sad to leave my safe haven. As I said my final goodbyes I turned my face away, leaving the horror of my tragedy behind. Looking ahead into the sunlight I knew I was ready to begin a new life.

...People look at the outer appearance,
but the Lord looks at the heart.

1 SAMUEL 16:7

CHAPTER TWELVE

On the ride home, so many different emotions ran through me: joyfulness, exhilaration, apprehension. I had driven home many times before on FDR Drive but now the experience seemed completely different. I looked at things with a new set of eyes, (unclear, damaged eyes.) I could not make out shapes unless sunlight was shining directly on them.

Along the way Mom and Dad pointed out certain buildings. When we approached the building in which I once worked, Mom said excitedly, "Mi-Mi, we are going past the Waffle Building. Look to your right and see if you can see it." I stared intently out the window. A building appeared quickly. Dad tried to slow down so I could get a better glimpse of it. I only saw the outline of the building with little squares. I frowned with frustration. I blinked a few times hoping it would clear my vision but it did nothing. Looking out the front windshield I thought I could make out the outline of the Brooklyn Bridge. I gasped, pointed, and shouted, "Is that the Brooklyn Bridge?"

Mom and Dad responded in unison "Yes!" Mom enthusiastically asked, "Can you see it clearly?" I squinted trying to focus.

Sadly I replied, "No. I can only see the outline. I can't tell if there are any cars on it or not." I sat back feeling troubled with my eye situation. We were all trying to figure out how much vision I had, since it fluctuated from day to day and moment to moment. None of us understood how much damage the TEN (toxic epidermal necrolysis) had done to my eyes. Exhausted I curled up on the back seat. A thousand thoughts raced through my mind. I made a promise to myself that restoring my eyesight would be my priority over anything else. Feeling reassured, I closed my eyes allowing sleep to come.

I awoke to Mom's gentle voice calling my name. We had arrived. We lived in a beautiful central-hall colonial house. My bedroom was on the second floor. Paulette and I shared a room. Temporarily I would be sleeping in my grandparents' room on the first floor. They had gone to live with my aunt since Mom couldn't care for them when I was in the hospital. I felt extremely guilty about that. I hoped one day when I felt better they would come back to live with us.

As Mom helped me out of the car I felt strangely nervous. I looked around trying to focus on my surroundings. I looked towards the garage and saw this incredible electric blue color. I fixed my eyes on it. It suddenly registered in my brain that it was my car. I yelled out with delight, "Is that my car?! Ma, please help me walk over to it." Tears streamed down my face; I was overwhelmed with emotions. I leaned my forehead against the edge of the roof and cried. I placed my hand on it feeling the shape of it. My heart ached realizing I wouldn't be able to drive it. I couldn't deal with the pain. I looked over at Mom and Dad. They were both crying. I asked them, "Can I please sit in it for a while? I need some time alone to sort out a few things in my heart and head."

Dad went into the house to get my keys. Mom hugged me. She repeated over and over, "Michelle, one day you will be driving it again. Have faith and never give up hope." I'm not sure how long I sat in the car. All I did was weep. My heart was broken for many reasons. Mom eventually came to get me. She gently opened the door and said, "Are you ready to come into the house?" I nodded. Slowly we walked towards the door. Mom reminded me of the large step. As we went up the step my legs gave out from underneath me and I fell to the ground. Mom almost came down with me. Mom shouted for Dad to come. She was scared I had hurt myself.

When Dad saw me crumpled on the ground he became alarmed. He looked at Mom and said, "What happened? She didn't see the step?"

Through Mom's sobs she said, "She put one leg up and when she went to lift the other leg, she collapsed. I guess her leg muscles aren't strong enough to go up a step."

I was dazed still trying to figure out what happened. Dad swooped me into his arms as if I was light as a feather. He gently placed me on the couch in the family room. Mom came over to check whether I was hurt. Thank God for no broken bones. Otherwise my homecoming would have been short-lived.

The doorbell rang as Mom prepared dinner. Instinctively I tried to get up to answer it. As I stood up I realized I was unsteady on my feet. I needed someone's support to help me walk. The kitchen was adjacent to the family room. When Mom saw me she freaked. She quickly came over to me and said, "Hold my arm. We will answer the door together."

It was Nick, Glenda, and the boys. I had not seen Nick since our little spat in the hospital. Everyone was happy to see me. When Nick hugged me he whispered, "I knew you could do it. Welcome home." When he pulled away from me I saw tears in his eyes. I never saw my brother so emotional in my life. My brothers were always so macho, strong, and tough. I smiled inwardly.

Nicholas and Michael pulled at my clothes yelling, "Aunt Mi-Mi! Aunt Mi-Mi!" I looked down at them, noticing Michael was no longer afraid of me. I wondered why. Was it because I was at home in regular clothing? I wanted so badly to pick them up and shower kisses all over them just like I used to. I couldn't; I was too weak. The boys wanted to help me back to the couch. I froze, knowing I needed more help than their two little hands. Mom noticed my hesitation. She came over and held my upper arm. "You hold their hands and I will hold you." My heart soared with joy. How I loved this mother of mine.

Paulette came home from work. She had no idea I would be home. Mom wanted to surprise her. Paulette had only come once to the hospital. She couldn't deal with what had happened to me. When she saw me she hugged me tight, and in between her sobs she apologized for not coming to the hospital more often. She told me she thought about me and prayed for me every day. I understood. I had no ill feelings towards her. I imagined this tragedy was life-altering for her as well. She was my baby sister. She had always looked up to me wanting my protection.

Mom made an incredible dinner. Everyone loved the food and had a good time. They were all laughing, debating, joking at the dinner table. The noise level was high and so were our spirits—your typical Italian family dinner—just as I remembered. Sometimes I felt a little overwhelmed and out of place. I had been confined to a hospital room for the past three and a half months. The only noise came from the medical equipment or the low voices of the patients and staff. I needed to adjust to this way of living again.

I was a little tired from all of the activities of the day. I had a few embarrassing moments at the dinner table. Mom put a cutlet on my plate. I had just learned how to hold a fork in my right hand. My left hand was weaker than my right so I wasn't able to hold any silverware in that hand. In the hospital Mom had cut all my food. I sat there in a panic. I didn't want anyone to see my imperfections. She was busy serving everyone. I didn't want to act like a child and ask her to cut my meat. I just sat there contemplating what to do. When Mom finally sat down to eat she noticed I wasn't eating. She asked from across the table, "Mi-Mi, what is wrong? Are you not hungry? It's your favorite, veal cutlets." Tears pricked the back of my eyes. Everyone was quiet and looking at me. My face reddened. I hung my head.

With all the dignity left in me I said in a small voice, "I am not capable of cutting my meat."

Mom sprung out of her seat shouting, "O Dio mio, I forgot! I am so sorry. I was doing a million things at once." Suddenly I had three sets of hands wanting to help me.

The other incident occurred when I reached for my glass. It was heavier than I expected. It wobbled in my hand spilling its contents on the table. Again everyone came to my rescue. This time tears trickled down my face. I felt totally humiliated. I had interrupted everyone's dinner twice. I felt like a big burden. I was relieved when dinner was over and everyone went home.

As Mom prepared my bed the phone rang. It was David. I had been waiting all night for his call. Our conversation was brief. He sensed I was exhausted from the day's events. He promised to call the following night and come to see me over the weekend. That was only four days away but it would seem like a lifetime. Mom helped me walk to my new room. As we got closer I remembered the doors to my grandparents' bedroom were mirrored. My heart quickened. I wasn't sure if I had the courage to look at myself in the mirror.

I abruptly stopped walking. "Mom, can you please turn off the light in the foyer? I don't want to see my reflection. I'm just not ready." Mom frowned. She began to say something but thought better not to. Reluctantly she nodded her head, understanding my insecurity. We entered the room. I looked around trying to focus, familiarizing myself with my new room. Everything seemed odd. I wondered if this is how prisoners felt when they got out of prison.

I sat on the bed. It was so comfortable, unlike the hospital beds. Mom handed me my pajamas. I looked at them as if they were a foreign object. I had worn a hospital gown for the past three and a half months. Would I feel constricted wearing them? I was tired and overthinking everything. Once settled in bed I realized the pillows were the ones from the hospital. I laughed and asked Mom, "Did you take the pillows from the hospital?"

She chuckled. "The nurses gave them to me to take home. You told them how comfortable they were. They wanted you to sleep well." Mom leaned over and kissed me good night. Before she left she said, "I am glad you are home. Remember, don't get up from the bed on your own or try to walk by yourself. Wait for me. If you need me just holler. My door will be open. I will see you in the morning. Sleep well. I love you."

I couldn't fall asleep. It was very dark and too quiet. I was accustomed to all kinds of sounds during the night in the hospital. I lay there terrified. My heart thumped in my chest. My breathing became labored. Frightening thoughts cluttered my mind. I sat up in bed. I wasn't sure how much time had passed since Mom left. I tried to reach for the lamp switch beside my bed and accidently I knocked over the glass of water on the nightstand. I panicked. I didn't know what to do. I grabbed some clothing from inside the night table to dry up the water. I continued to look for the light switch and couldn't find it. I finally gave up.

I began to cry out for Mom. My cries went unheard. My chest hurt. I couldn't breathe properly. I was having a panic attack. Getting on my hands and knees I crawled to the bedroom door. I screamed out loudly with all the breath I had left. Mom finally heard me. The sound of my pounding heart roared in my ears. I barely heard her footsteps coming down the stairs. Mom took me into her arms and held me. Helping take control of my breathing, she said "Michelle, focus on me. It's time to smell the roses. Take a deep breath in, in, in, and let it out. Follow my breathing." I focused, listening to Mom's directions. After a long while I relaxed. My breathing went back to normal. Mom helped me to my feet and back into bed. She sat beside me and asked, "What happened?" ashamed of myself I admitted, "I was afraid to be down here by myself. My mind was playing tricks on me and I began to get nervous. I tried to turn on the light and I knocked over the water. I made a mess."

Worried, Mom took my hand and said, "Do you want me to sleep in the room with you until you feel comfortable sleeping on your own?" I looked up at her with love and admiration.

I answered softly, "You wouldn't mind doing that? It will make me feel better if you did."

Mom smiled and said, "It's no problem. I will sleep with you however long it takes. I will do anything for you. Let me clean this up and let's get some sleep. We have a busy day tomorrow."

I squeezed her hand. "I love you Ma. Thank you for everything."

The following days and weeks indeed proved to be busy. My wheelchair, oxygen tank, and shower chair were delivered. Phone calls were made arranging physical therapy, occupational therapy, doctor appointments, and so on. Calls came in from different organizations, social workers, and friends who wanted to visit. My excitement about being home grew each day.

Realizing how much I had to do, I set priorities. First, feel better and become stronger physically; second, adjust to being at home; third, find an ophthalmologist who specialized in corneal disease and who was familiar with TEN; and fourth, get another opinion on the severity of my condition, and how to restore my eyesight.

Being home I faced new challenges each day. Routine things I once did so easily and gracefully were now very difficult and awkward. Taking a shower was a problem. I was accustomed to showering in a larger area in the hospital; at home it was more of a confined area. I felt claustrophobic. Old fears resurfaced. Mom always sensed my anxiety. She took control of the situation and put me at ease. She came into the shower in her undergarments and gave me a hand with whatever I needed. When we were done she would assist me into the wheelchair, guide me into my room, help me dry myself, and put my clothes on. I felt like a child. I wondered if I would ever be able to do anything for myself again and live a normal life.

Friends from high school took turns visiting me. I hesitated to let myself be seen in this condition. I felt insecure about how I appeared. I was extremely nervous they would judge me for what I looked like on the outside forgetting I was still the same Michelle on the inside. It was important for me to maintain my circle of friends so I could have some sort of a social life outside of my family. My fears turned out to be justified. Some of my so-called friends came to visit and never returned or contacted me again. I felt like a freak in a circus act, a spectacle. Did they come over only to satisfy their curiosity? It was certainly not to give me moral support. They hurt me deeply. The only friends who remained loyal were Stacie, Christine, Maria, Joanne, Johnny, and Sal.

I continued to repair my broken life putting aside the emotional hurt, trying to strengthen my physical being. Meanwhile depression lurked around me. I constantly battled to keep it away. I would never surrender to it. I tried to keep my spirits up by spending time with my true friends, my loving family, and of course David who called me each night.

My first weekend home, David broke his promise. He didn't come to visit. He explained he wanted to give me time with my family and adjust to my new way of life. I was very upset with his decision. I didn't understand or agree with him. I was eager to see him and spend a little time alone with him. I had no choice but to accept it. I wanted to maintain some kind of normalcy in this chaotic life.

I worked hard with my physical therapist to regain my strength. I made small improvements each day. As I became steadier on my feet my physical therapist taught me little tricks so I would rely less on anyone's help. I could walk independently with a little assistance from a wall or by pushing a wheelchair. My grip grew stronger too. I constantly had a therapy ball in my hands to strengthen my muscles.

I learned not to rely heavily on the little bit of eyesight that I had when eating. They taught me to use my plate like a clock, the top being twelve o'clock, bottom being six o'clock; the right and left sides were three and nine o'clock. This would help me to know where Mom placed my food and what food was in those time zones. In some of my training sessions Mom had to be with me in order for her to know how to make things easier for me. This was all new to both of us so we eagerly learned together. Mom expressed pride in my accomplishments, acting like my personal cheerleader as she still is today. I strived each day to do more. I was anxious to recapture my old life.

The second weekend passed with no visit from David. Once again he gave me a number of reasons why he couldn't come. This time he had to be at the office preparing for year-end work but he promised to definitely come the following week. I thought it to be a little odd he was working this early in the month on year-end stuff. My spirits declined. With words unuttered I began to have this sick feeling in my gut. I prayed the unspoken would not happen between David and me. I held onto whatever was left of my determination, and moved forward with my life. I worked hard, convincing myself the next time I saw David I would show him how far I had come from the days of being confined to a hospital bed. I would make him proud of me with how soon things would be back to normal. (That way of thinking would give me the renewed energy I needed until the next weekend.)

Just when I thought nothing else could be taken away from me physically, emotionally, and spiritually, the unspoken happened. Another weekend passed and no David. He called but this phone call was like no other. His words cut through my heart slowly, deeply, and painfully. I heard only phrases... he was leaving me...ending the relationship...couldn't continue to lie...no longer pretending everything was all right between us...couldn't handle a relationship with me anymore...wanted to remain friends...wanted to call me periodically to see how I was doing. I listened in total shock. I couldn't believe what he was saying. Unbearable pain sliced through my body. All those promises he'd made, were they lies? Was it merely guilt? Treating me like an object of pity? In the hospital every night before he left he told me he'd never leave me, saying, "I will always be by your side; I'm stuck on you just like peanut butter sticks to the roof of your mouth." I held the phone in my hand, as raw, bitter, humiliating betrayal seized me. Scalding, angry tears spilled down my face. I demanded answers from him. "Did you lie to me? Did you come to the hospital only because you felt sorry for me?"

David defended himself and his motives but it sounded like a weak, vain attempt to reassure me. I couldn't believe him. Unable to handle the torturous pain anymore I ended the call by telling him loudly, "I never want to see you again! And don't contact me ever again!" Devastated, I hung up. I sat at the kitchen table in disbelief, feeling sick to my stomach. How was I going to tell Mom and everyone else what he just did to me? I couldn't tell her the truth; she would hunt him down and tear him to shreds.

I had to think quick. I heard Mom's footsteps approaching. She must have heard me shouting at David. Unprepared for her questioning I sat there silently. She sat down beside me. Taking my hands into hers, she asked tenderly, "What was that all about? Why did you tell him never to call you again? Did you have a fight with him because he didn't come see you?"

I hung my head. I didn't have the courage to look at her. My heart was in pieces. With tears spilling down my face, I contemplated a fraction of a second whether to tell Mom the truth about David. At first I thought if I confided in her, she could help me heal, as her strength would help me through this painful time. But on second thought I decided it would be best to endure this alone. I looked into Mom's eyes and told her the half-truth, "I ended my relationship with David. I asked him never to call or see me again." I had just lied to my beautiful mother, the woman who had sacrificed her life for me.

Mom's eyes grew round in disbelief. Astounded, she asked me, "Why did you do that? You need his support more than ever during this time." I just sat there in despair. Mom shook my hands vigorously as if to wake me up. "Why did you do that to him? He came every night when you were in the coma. How could you hurt him? You need to call him back and apologize. Tell him you were angry because he broke his promises the last few weeks." Tears were now falling down Mom's face too.

I couldn't believe I was hurting the person I loved the most and who loved me more than anyone on earth. I didn't know what to do or say to make her feel better. Softly I managed, "I am not going to call him back. He needs to move on with his life. It's unfair for him to get stuck with a girlfriend in my condition. I'm not even a woman anymore. Look at me. He deserves better!" I couldn't believe what was coming out of my mouth. Why was I protecting David? Did I hope he would come back to me? I didn't want anyone to have ill feelings towards him. Mom was extremely angry at me. She stalked away, crying. Now my heart bled from two wounds: one from David for betraying me and the other for betraying Mom.

Despair made me turn inward. I was lifeless. Bleak darkness and unhappiness were running through my veins. I no longer wanted to live this horrible life that was now mine. I increasingly became despondent and depressed. I slowly regressed. All I did was lie in bed in a fetal position hoping for the pain to go away. I was angry at God for everything that had happened to me. I was also angry with Mom who had made me live, since I no longer wanted to live this miserable existence-of-mine. I withdrew from everyone and everything. I stopped eating properly. I gave up on my physical therapy, hoping my body would just wither away. I don't know how long I remained this way—days, weeks, I'm not sure.

Mom's worry increased each day that passed. Deep, deep inside I knew I couldn't reach out to Mom. She was begging me to call David so I could end my suffering. I wanted to shout out: *David is the one who left me! He is the reason I am going through this! He doesn't want me anymore!* Mom didn't understand. This wasn't only about David, but also what had become of me.

I felt alone and abandoned. I was broken. I had reached bottom. I had been reduced to nothing and yet, here I was, still breathing. I wondered why. In my deep despair I searched for something. Returning to my faith I prayed to God for strength and a reason to live. My answer was right in front of me. I had to live for my Mom. She had sacrificed so much of her life for me. Giving up and willing myself to die would be selfish on my part. It would kill her if anything happened to me. During my coma, I'd had a vision. I could jump into the abyss or I could choose to live. During this vision I was even closer to death but was still offered a choice. Jesus sent me back to my Mother. At that moment I made the decision life was worth living. If a shattered person like me could be offered a choice to live as if she was a precious gift of God, who was I to deny it? Since I had been given a second chance I would be thankful and live life to its fullest regardless of all of my new challenges. This was the turning point of my life.

I never shared with anyone the truth about David. I suffered in silence. I told everyone the same story over and over, that I had been the one to break up with him. Family and friends thought I was courageous and selfless to set him free. Each time they said something like that, I felt guilty. But I knew inwardly this was best. If they had known the truth, they would have been out for blood. They were all very protective of me. Today, I truly believe that by telling everyone I was the one to end the relationship it helped heal my broken heart by avoiding the reality of David's hurtful rejection so I could move on with my life.

The next four years were very busy. I continued with physical therapy for several years. Slowly I became more active even though I still had a lot of health issues. One good memory I have is when Nick picked me up from physical therapy on his motorcycle. I was thrilled to go for a ride. I asked him "Does Mommy know you are taking me home on the motorcycle?"

He laughed. "No. Are you crazy? She would have yelled at me. She will know when we get there." Laughing with him I excitedly hopped on the bike. The ride was exhilarating. When we arrived home we both felt guilty and nervous just like two little kids who did something wrong. I skulked into the house with the helmet under my arm. Mom stood in the kitchen preparing dinner. She turned to look at me and her mouth dropped. She stood there stunned. (It is at your own risk to approach Mom in the kitchen especially if it isn't about something good. She always had some kind of utensil in her hand and you never knew what she would do with it.) I laughed at her reaction. I knew I wouldn't catch Mom's wrath. Nick would be seen as the one responsible. But he was smart and stayed outside waiting for us, hoping Mom wouldn't make a scene in front of the neighbors.

Hesitantly Mom asked me, "You're joking, right? Nick didn't bring you home on the motorcycle?"

Smiling ear-to-ear I said, "It's not a joke. The motorcycle is outside. Don't be mad. It was fun. I loved it."

In a swift instant she went outside with her utensil in her hand. Laughing, I followed her outside, pleading with her to have mercy on Nick. Nick has always been a good sport. He was a mischievous child and teenager. He was always in trouble (and if he wasn't, he knew how to find it.) He knew how to handle Mom. We always said, "Nick has her wrapped around his little finger." He helped me immensely during my recovery. If I couldn't do something or just gave up, he inspired me to continue or he would find a way it was easier for me. The words "I can't do it" did not exist in Nick's vocabulary.

One day we went to Nick and Glenda's house. There were twenty steps up before reaching the door. During this time I was still weak and having difficulty going up steps. After trying several times I gave up. Nick put me on piggyback, and up-the-stairs we went. When we reached the landing he said, "One day you will be able to do that on your own." He was right. I am now going up and down stairways in my heels with no problems at all.

Finding an ophthalmologist was very challenging. In 1986 the internet was not in every home. I made phone call after phone call to different hospitals and eye infirmaries throughout the country. Thank heavens, I found a brilliant doctor who specialized in TEN at the New York Eye and Ear Infirmary.

The chase to regain my eyesight began in the spring of 1987. At this point my little bit of vision worsened considerably. My eyelids had stuck to my eyeballs, not allowing me to open my eyelids properly. Continuous surgeries were done to reverse the damage from TEN. The first week I had four eye surgeries back-to-back every day. If the doctors were successful I would be able to see somewhat clearly. On the last day the doctors had trouble waking me up from the anesthesia. One of the fellow doctors frantically went searching for Mom. He knew I was on a specific breathing medication but it wasn't listed on my chart. He found Mom in my room praying. Breathlessly he asked Mom, "Mrs. Frazzetto, I need to know, what breathing medicine does Michelle take?"

Mom looked at him in a panic and said, "What's wrong? Is Michelle OK? Is she out of surgery?"

The doctor looked at Mom and firmly said, "I will explain everything to you, but I need to know the name of the medicine."

Stricken, Mom said, "She is on Theo-Dur." Immediately the doctor called down to the operating room, giving them the information. The difficult part for him now was explaining to Mom what had happened. Gesturing for Mom to sit, he calmly began to explain. Fear and worry overwhelmed Mom. In a panic she leaped off the seat, rushing out of the room trying to get to me. The doctor grabbed Mom's arm to stop her. He gently told her, "Mrs. Frazzetto, they won't let you into Recovery. In a few minutes I will call down to see how Michelle is doing. If they have stabilized her I will take you to see her. In the meantime I will stay here with you."

This doctor was our favorite. He was always so warm and kind with us. Finally they allowed Mom to come. Her heart tore in two when she saw me. I lay there asleep. I had a patch over my left eye. My face was very pale. Mom couldn't contain her tears. She just didn't understand why I had to go through more suffering. Anger gripped her.

Leaving the recovery room in desperation she went to the nearby church. Questioning her faith, she stormed through the church doors, her heart black as coal. Angrily she walked up the center aisle towards the statue of Jesus. Throwing her fists in the air she shouted to the statue, "Why? Why is this happening to my daughter? She never did anything wrong to anyone! Why are you doing this to her?" Before Mom said something she would regret, she passed out, falling to the floor. When she awoke she was lying on the church bench. People surrounded her, trying to wake her up. Feeling utterly ashamed and guilty for her anger towards Jesus she began to weep. Mom sat there for a long time, repenting and praying to God for forgiveness.

Mom and I both were rewarded for our endurance the next day when my bandage was removed. Anxious to see what the results were, my heart pounded in my chest. My doctors asked me to play a little game with them. Since I had no idea what any of the doctors looked like, they asked me to pick who was who as they sat in complete silence. In my mind I had envisioned what they looked like according to their voice.

Gently the doctor began to remove the tape that held the bandage in place. I could feel my heart quicken with each passing moment. When the bandage was finally removed my heart stopped. My eye was closed shut. I could tell the room was dark. Saline drops were squirted on the eyelid to soften the dried blood from the surgery. Gently the doctor wiped the eyelid clean. A slit lamp was placed in front of me, so I could place my chin on it. Slowly the doctor cleaned the eyelashes with a sterile swab. With another sterile swab the doctor carefully began to lift my eyelid open. I took in a sharp breath with surprise when color and shapes came into view. It was the most incredible, exhilarating feeling in the world. The only way I can describe that moment and what I saw is when the movie "The Wizard of Oz" goes from black and white into color.

From my reaction the doctor knew I could see. Pulling the slit-lamp away from me, he stood up and went to stand with the other two doctors. I anxiously turned my head looking for my Mom. There she was. Her face was as beautiful as I remembered it. Tears of joy trickled down her face. I stared at her in disbelief. I extended my hand to touch her face and said, "Ma, you look the same. You haven't changed at all. You are still beautiful." She rubbed her face against my hand. Love and happiness filled our hearts.

I turned to look at the doctors. It was time to play their little game. The brilliant doctor who had performed the surgery was the oldest. He was the easiest to pick out. The other two were fairly young. One was tall, slender, and really good looking. The other was shorter and not so handsome. One of them had an incredibly sexy voice with a slight accent. So I assumed that belonged to the tall, hot doctor. The other doctor had a soft, melodic voice so I assumed that belonged to the other. Watching the confusion on my face, the not-so-handsome doctor said, "I am Dr. D." (He was the doctor with the sexy voice. I crinkled my nose in disappointment.) I quickly looked over at the other doctor. In a sing-song I-am-in-love-with-you voice, I purred, "You must be Dr. Lister." The entire room erupted in laughter. Dr. Lister is still my surgeon as well as a close friend of mine. I still have a secret crush on him after all these years. (Oops, I guess the secret is out.)

On the very same day I found the courage to finally look at myself in the mirror. I didn't know what to expect; I had not seen myself in many months. My face felt thin and my scars felt hideous; the thought made me nervous and anxious. I shared my thought with Mom as we went back to my room. She told me, "I will be here with you whatever you decide." Mom's support was all I needed. We both stood a few feet away from the mirror. My heart pounded in my chest; my body trembled. Mom took my hand in hers, assuring me, "Michelle, you have nothing to be afraid of. You are still beautiful. Come closer to the mirror to see for yourself."

I slowly approached the mirror. Suddenly, my reflection came into view. I looked at myself wide-eyed in surprise. My face didn't look horrible at all. I looked slightly different. My facial features were more pronounced because I was thin. The color and style of my hair and the shape of my eyes were not the same. I no longer had my beautiful eyes and my hair was short and dark brown.

Transfixed on my facial reflection at first, I finally looked away not having the courage to look at my scars. I knew I had to face them. Gathering strength, I took a deep breath to calm my pounding heart. Tears pooled in my eyes. Looking at myself once again I slowly brought my gaze downward towards my upper chest. A thousand emotions hit me at once…hurt, anger, self-pity. The scars were ugly. They were raised, and glowed bright pink. I hated them. They were on a part of a woman's body that was so important, the décolletage. Every time I looked into a mirror I would have to see scars. Abruptly

I turned away. I couldn't believe the change in me. I would not allow what I just witnessed to kill my spirits. Instead, I focused on the happiness Mom and I felt with the outcome of the eye surgery. I got into bed more determined than ever. I would work hard to reverse all the damage of TEN.

Throughout the years to follow I went to see several reconstructive surgeons. It entailed many complicated and intense surgeries, with no guarantee of leaving any residual scars, and it wasn't a chance I was willing to take. Embarrassed about them, I hid them with my clothing for many years. Today I have a different attitude about them. I wear my scars proudly. I am no longer ashamed of them.

Our joy was short-lived. After several months my body began to reject the cornea and it became opaque, making it impossible to see clearly anymore. Throughout the twenty-seven years, multiple surgeries were performed in my left eye. I kept track of how many surgeries by keeping the hospital bracelets. After collecting one hundred of them I stopped. With each bracelet I saved, I hoped that it was going to be the last, or "the lucky one." There was never a lucky one; yet, I never gave up. I always lived with the hope to see one day. In my right eye I had some functional vision. The right eye rarely had any surgeries. In the ophthalmology world you only did surgery on one eye at a time preserving the other eye for any future possibilities for perfect vision.

Mom and I took a trip to Italy to see Teresa. It was a much-needed vacation for both of us. The last time I had seen Teresa was in the intensive care unit the previous year. It was great to be with my nieces, relatives, and Italian friends.

We returned to Italy three years later. We went to see a doctor in Rome. The city of Rome was one of the places I had not visited on my prior trips to Italy but I had promised myself to go one day. I never imagined it would be with no sight. This doctor was working on a device for eyes with damaged surfaces and corneas. I was excited to explore my option of regaining my eyesight, and sad because I no longer had any vision to see all the beauty the city had to offer. (I had unexpectedly lost the little bit of functional vision in my right eye due to a perforation of the cornea. I only had light perception and I could see colors.) The Roman doctor's device turned out to be not an option for me. It would be absolutely hideous. They had to remove the entire front of the eye, pupil, iris, et cetera. Then they would cover the entire eye with mucus membrane taken from my mouth. A tube made from my tooth would be placed in the center of the eye which would allow me to see through it. I made the decision to remain the way I was rather than look at myself in that horrific way.

My pursuit of regaining my eyesight never ended. I became obsessed with wanting to see again. I traveled to Spain, Boston, Louisiana, Kentucky, and Florida. The hope and desire to see again fueled my determination to continue to live. Without that hope constantly in my life, I would have given up.

In 1989 my parents and I went on vacation to Florida to look for a place where Dad could retire. Sal and Jeanette were now married and living there. They had visited a quaint town on the west coast while honeymooning. Mom and Dad wanted to explore it for themselves. They fell in love with it immediately. They decided to put the New York house up for sale. They thought it would take a year or so to sell, giving me some time to accept their decision to move. I was extremely unhappy with this sudden change. The thought of relocating to Florida made me nervous. My life finally had become somewhat normal. I didn't want any disruptions; I'd had so many of them in the recent past. The thought of leaving behind my friends, family, and everything I-loved-and-knew caused me anxiety. My biggest fear was leaving Dr. Lister, my eye doctor. He was the only doctor I trusted to do my surgeries. I was also worried about living in an area that I never saw and wasn't familiar with: streets, stores, doctor's offices, and so on.

We were all very surprised and unprepared when the house sold four months later. I no longer had the luxury of time to accept Mom and Dad's decision. The reality of it was only a few months away. I became depressed. I had ideas about getting my own place and remaining on Staten Island. I knew that wasn't a possibility for many reasons. For one, Mom certainly wouldn't leave me behind. I still wasn't completely healthy and I only had light-perception, not true vision in either eye. I wouldn't be able to take care of myself and didn't want to be a burden to my brother and his family. My resources were limited. Even Paulette and her new husband had moved to Florida.

Knowing I had no other choice I decided to go along with my parents who had sacrificed their lives for me. I prayed heart and soul for acceptance, guidance, and serenity.

Moving day arrived. Heading south on I-95 I sat in the back seat of my parents' car gazing at the sunlight from the passenger window. I had many thoughts and mixed emotions. Although I had come to terms with the fact of moving, it still was extremely difficult leaving behind the place I grew up and lived all of my life. It had been painful to say goodbye to my closest friends and family. With a single tear slowly streaming down my face I wondered if it was a tear of joy for the beginning of my new life or a tear of sorrow for the old life I was leaving behind. Perhaps it was a tear for both. After so many sleepless nights I had found a silver lining. I would be moving to a place where no one knew me and couldn't judge me for what I looked like. I no longer had to endure secret whispers and comments from relatives and acquaintances on how I had changed, always comparing the person I had been with the person I had become. It was like a second chance. Any new person I met would only know the Michelle I was today, and not the Michelle I once was. They wouldn't know my hair had once been blonde and not light brown. They wouldn't know I had not been blind four years prior. No one would know I was much thinner now. They would just accept and love me for who I was today.

The thought was refreshing. I finally would be free to be me! Michelle! On that long trip from New York to Florida I allowed these thoughts to soothe my soul and bring peace to my heart. I knew no matter what, everything was going to be OK. I would be with the two people who loved me more than their own lives, and I would be free to create my own life under their loving care. That was something that would never change.

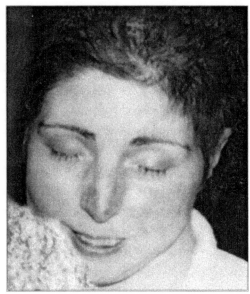

*Three months after coming home from the hospital,
the eyelids had adhered to the eyes*

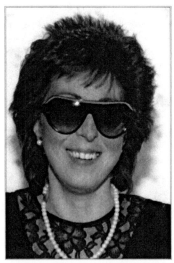

After One Year

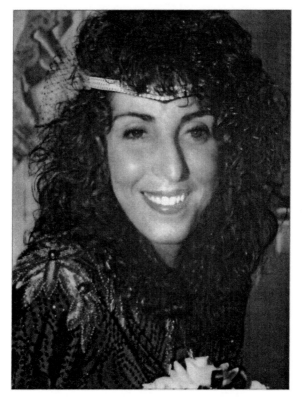

After Two Years

I know what it is to be in need, and know what it is to have plenty. I have learned the secret of being content ...I can do everything through him who gives me strength. Yet it was good of you to share in my troubles...

PHILIPPIANS 4:12-14

EPILOGUE:
MY RAINBOW AFTER THE STORM

My first several years in Florida were filled with new and interesting experiences. Coming from New York where everything and everyone moved at a fast pace, our Florida city seemed extremely laid back, and moved at a turtle's speed. No one rushed on the roads or in the stores. The majority of people spoke with a southern accent and extended their warm, friendly hospitality.

We rented a house for a few months until my parents' new home was finished. Mom and Dad's house was absolutely beautiful with three bedrooms, three bathrooms, formal living and dining rooms, and an in-ground swimming pool and spa. Mom and Dad were always thoughtful and considerate of my needs. They made the second bedroom into my personal den for entertaining friends. They added a door sectioning off my space allowing me some privacy. My bedroom had french doors which opened onto the lanai by the pool area. Simply paradise!

We spent our days exploring, acclimating ourselves to the area. I also spent a lot of time with Paulette and her husband. I met new people and made friends through their social circles.

Before moving to Florida I had decided to fly back to New York every three months to see Dr. Lister. In Florida I also searched for an ophthalmologist nearby who would be familiar with my eye condition. I settled on a doctor who had heard of TEN but did not specialize in it. He agreed to check my eyes at least monthly to make sure everything remained stable. He was neglectful by not doing glaucoma screening, and between visits to New York I developed complications in my right eye. It was devastating. I had to let the Florida doctor go. (Fortunately, years later, I found an outstanding corneal specialist who is dedicated to my care, and monitors me closely.)

Due to the seriousness of the situation, Dr. Lister and a glaucoma specialist immediately performed eye surgery. They placed a shunt and a corneal graft trying to save the eye. Unfortunately because of the first Florida doctor's negligence, the glaucoma had destroyed most of the optic nerve. A post-operative infection did further damage. Dr. Lister had a very difficult time telling me that the damage to my eye was irreversible. I grieved deeply for months. It was like a death. My hopes of ever seeing out of the right eye were gone forever; another tragic loss in my life.

After moving into the new house I had considered whether to attend the local school for the blind. The school taught visually impaired people and blind people to live independently. At first I was reluctant because in my heart of hearts I still hoped I would see one day. Going to the blind school would imply I was giving up and accepting my blindness. After many weeks of discussing it with Mom and Dad I finally relented and went to the school. It was definitely a learning experience. I was the youngest in my class. Everyone was at least two generations older. After the second week I didn't want to return. I had nothing in common with any of my classmates. They had lost their sight due to old age or diabetes. I just didn't fit in. Besides, Mom was the best teacher. She had taught me so much in the four years since my accident. Time after time Mom encouraged me to go back to the school and continue to learn. Today I am glad I did. They showed me different techniques on how to cook and iron safely. They also taught me how to fold my paper money and how to tell the difference between coins. They always emphasized how we must focus and visualize everything we were doing, and not to rely on the little bit of vision we may have had. I also took classes in computer and Braille. Walking with a white cane was the last part of my training. My heart tore into pieces during these sessions. I deeply suffered emotionally to have to walk with a cane. It was something I just could not accept and still can't today. A helping arm is always available from my family and my devoted friends. I call all of them "my seeing eye angels."

The pot of gold at the end of the rainbow was Scott, an incredible guy whom I met several months after relocating. Scott brought all the colors of the rainbow back into my life. His heart was warm, kind, caring, and generous. We fell instantly in love. Scott gave me the piece of the puzzle that was missing in my heart and life. Until this point I had only been existing and not living. Scott overlooked all of my imperfections. He appreciated my intelligence and wit, and made me feel beautiful once again. He never saw me as a blind girl. Scott made me do and try everything for the first time as a sightless person. We traveled. We took college classes together. He took me jet-skiing, boating, horseback riding, bowling, miniature golfing, working out in a gym, four-wheeling, and all of life's other fun things.

After being together five years Scott and I became engaged. One year later we built a home together around the corner from my Mom and Dad's. It was extremely difficult moving out of my parent's house. Actually, I didn't move out for a while; I moved out by degrees. I lived with my parents four days a week and in my new home the other three days. After a few months of doing that, Mom sat me down to talk. She was gentle with me. "Michelle, you have your own house now. It is time for you to make your house into a home. It will make me happy knowing you can live independently when the day arrives and I'm no longer here with you."

Unhappiness filled my heart. "Are you throwing me out? I can't leave the dogs!"

Mom laughed. "Of course I'm not throwing you out. If it were up to me, I would baby you for the rest of my life. This is hard for me too. But I know I have to let you go and spread your wings. As for Shayna and Bianca, they can have sleepovers anytime you want." We hugged tightly as tears of joy streamed down our faces. It was the wisest advice Mom had ever given me.

Today I live independently. I cook, clean, do my wash, iron, and even take out the garbage. Visitors always have two questions: "Who cleans your house? It is immaculate and spotless!" and "Who decorated your home? It's absolutely beautiful."

Laughing with pride I say, "I clean my own house and I did all the decorating myself with a little help. I tell the person-I'm-shopping-with what I envision in my mind's eye. When they find what I want, they describe it to me as I feel the object with my hands."

I choose and buy my clothing the same way. I tell whomever I'm shopping with what I am looking for. They leave me at the clothing rack. When I feel the style of something interesting, I try to see the color. I pick it up, asking my friend or family member to describe it fully to me. I do wear quite a bit of black. Don't worry—it is always sleek and classy! My nurse would be proud.

After four years of living together Scott literally distanced himself from me. He had a new job in which he traveled a lot. He was gone for months. When he was absent I stayed busy helping Mom with Dad's care. Dad had been diagnosed two years before with lung cancer and was slowly declining each month. Scott just grew in another direction, being away from me. When Scott broke up with me and permanently moved out, my world turned upside down. I had been so consumed with Dad's health I never saw the break-up coming. The shock totally devastated me and hurt me right to the core of my being. Once again the man I loved was leaving me at a time when I needed him most. I suffered in silence not wanting to burden Mom and Dad with my pain. The break-up seemed unimportant compared to what we were going through with Dad's terminal illness. I couldn't share my pain with them; they already had so much going on in their lives. They were also very hurt and upset with what happened; they loved Scott like a son.

I dedicated all of myself to Dad's comfort and care trying to put aside my personal hurt. Dad died six months after Scott left me. I miss my Dad every day. My heart aches with the emptiness. He certainly was an incredibly strong man to endure what he did. He fought long and hard to stay alive. He didn't want to leave me and Mom alone. Mom and I had each other during this difficult time just like always.

Thirteen years have passed since Scott and I separated. Although the break-up had almost destroyed me I hold no ill feelings towards Scott. After many months of healing my heart, remarkably I found forgiveness for him. I came to the realization that it isn't another person who brings you happiness. Happiness is within yourself. Today Scott and I talk often. Scott is married, and occasionally we all go out together. If I ever need anything, Scott is there to give me a helping hand. After all these years he still encourages me to fulfill my dreams. One of my greatest wishes was to drive my Firebird again. Recently, he took me to an undeveloped part of town and let me drive it. The feeling was exhilarating. Simply awesome! It had been twenty-eight years since I last drove the "Blue Beauty." Scott survived the experience fearlessly. Thank God. (Don't worry readers; I didn't hit anyone or anything.) I embrace and thank Scott for the ten wonderful, beautiful years together. In essence he gave me my life back. Scott is very appreciative for everything I have done for him as well. He is grateful that I helped him change his life in a positive way and grow into the confident man he is today. We share a deep fondness and respect for each other.

My brother Nick, Glenda, and the boys moved to Florida one year after us. They added a new member to their family. Glenda had given birth to a little baby boy named Paul. Nicholas and Michael were happy to have a new brother. After seventeen years of marriage, Nick and Glenda divorced. Nick is now remarried. Nicholas and Michael are all grown up, married, and have children of their own. Paul is still a bachelor. Glenda lives with Nicholas in New York. She never remarried. She dedicated her life to raising the boys. Today she enjoys her days with her new granddaughter. My brother Sal and Jeanette are still living in Florida. They have two great kids, Sal Jr. and Ashley. My sister Paulette and her first husband divorced, and she is now remarried and has two wonderful children, a boy and a girl. My sister Teresa, Guido, and the girls moved to Florida in 2008. After living in Italy for thirty years they decided to relocate to the United States. Their daughters Jessica, Jennifer, and Janet have grown up to be lovely young women. Jennifer is married to a lawyer and lives in Boston. The other two girls are focused on their careers and living life to its fullest.

My sassy friend Stacie is still living on Staten Island. She married and divorced the guy I mentioned in Chapter Four. The doctors always told Stacie as a young adult that she wouldn't be able to have children. She was blessed with four: Nicole, the twins Danielle and Shannon, and Joseph. God indeed has a sense of humor. After divorcing her husband and while raising her kids, Stacie went to college part time to get a Masters Degree in General/Special Education. We are still the best of friends and we try to see each other once a year. When we are together it's as if we are still those young girls from long ago.

I am sure you are all wondering about my magnificent Mom. After Dad died she built a smaller home next door to their other house. At age sixty-nine she went for her driver's license for the first time in her life. Dad had been old-fashioned and never wanted her to drive. Several months after receiving her license, Mom was afflicted with the debilitating and painful disease rheumatoid arthritis. During this dark period of time our roles had switched. I dedicated my life to Mom just as she had done for me. I became Mom's caregiver. I took care of her with the same love and patience she had given me. Despite all of her health ailments Mom's fiery spirit lives on! Her days are busy and occupied with her new puppy, Shayla. Since we both live alone I go to have dinner with her almost every night. She is still cooking her delicious meals for me. When our friends come over to eat they say "Nonni your food is always so scrumptious. Why is it when we try to make it at home it doesn't taste the same? What is your secret?"

With a Mona Lisa smile on her face and a twinkle in her eyes she says, "My secret is: I cook with love."

Dear readers, living life after surviving TEN has certainly not been easy. The lingering effects debilitate me each and every day of my life. As I get older my health issues slowly worsen. I suffer severely with COPD and bronchiectasis due to the many weeks on the respirator and the puncturing of my left lung. My mucous membranes are damaged throughout my body. My salivary glands no longer function properly; I am not able to eat any dry foods such as bread, cookies, crackers, etc. without drinking something along with it. My fingernails and toenails never grew back; the nail beds were ruined when the skin was removed from my hands and when the booties were on my feet. My immune system is badly compromised, making me susceptible to germs and disease. I'm constantly fighting off some kind of virus or bacteria. All of my internal organs have been affected one way or another. I also suffer with cholesteatomas in my ears. It is an abnormal cyst-like growth which develops in the ear canal impairing my hearing. It is imperative that I have these removed nearly every month to prevent any hearing loss. The surface of my eyes as well as my tear ducts were destroyed. My surface is so fragile I am always on high alert for any defects and perforations. My eyes constantly hurt and sting. I continually put artificial tears and ointment throughout the day to keep them somewhat comfortable. I am blind with some light perception in my left eye which allows me to see the beautiful sunlight and colors if they are placed in front of my eye. I thank and praise God for that little bit I still have.

After this life-changing tragedy I have so much fear and anxiety about taking any prescription drugs that I will only take them when absolutely necessary. I mainly use alternative medicine: applied kinesiology, chiropractic care, periodic lymphatic and colonic decongestive treatments, acupuncture, and massage therapy. I try to eat healthy and exercise daily. I am overwhelmed with my everyday care at times. Many of my days of the week are spent in doctors' offices just to maintain my health. TEN has definitely impacted and transformed my life.

The road to a full life out in society hasn't always been smooth. I was not even aware that prejudice against the blind existed until I became sight-impaired. I have endured from all types of people a surprising amount of humiliation, criticism, and whispers, mostly in the form of judgmental comments. I am also aware when people stop or suddenly become silent when I approach. During these trying times I have turned to my faith and inner strength to hold my head up high. Moreover, I have been blessed with warm, kind people who cross my path each day. They admire, respect, and accept me for who I am. When I go to the local shops, clerks know me by name and are always eager to help me in any way they can. I have captured and touched many strangers' hearts with my incredible story. They are amazed about my strength, my gentle spirit, and my positive and outgoing personality, leaving them with a lasting impression of me. My life has been enriched with beautiful and loyal friends. They are always there for me with a helping hand and would do anything to make my life a little easier if they could. They truly love and accept me for me, Michelle. I am grateful and thankful for each and every one of them. I have also been blessed to be included in my brother-in-law Chris's company where I currently volunteer part-time. Volunteering diverts my attention from my health issues. It allows me to feel somewhat whole again; giving me a purpose for life, a true blessing.

Although this tragedy happened to me, there's beauty and joy and wonder in each day that awaits me. My mother, my friends, my inborn gifts of warmth, humor, and faith in God inspire and empower me to move forward and never give up. Family and friends have told me I have accomplished so much through the years. Personally, it didn't seem like accomplishments at all. I had to do it; I didn't have a choice. It was a matter of fighting and surviving TEN. I feel as if I must strive to become all I can be and achieve the full potential of the gifts I have been given.

I am not certain what lies ahead for me or where my future will take me. I only know, whatever it is or wherever it goes, I'll still be wearing my heels.

COLORBLIND

by Robert Kellum

If I were blind and couldn't see
What would color mean to me?
Would shades of red, or green, or blue,
Have any power to imbue

The feelings they invoke so now?
Or could such feelings still somehow,
Find color simply on their own,
In forms of vision not yet known?

Could I still feel blue's calming cold?
The warmth of red?, or yellow's bold?
What would an inner landscape mean,
Experiencing violet, or green?

What color the warmth of a noonday sun?
What color touch from a dear loved one?
What color, depths of passion stirred?
Of feeling valued, feeling heard?

What color crickets in spring night air?
Or the smell of a lover's perfumed hair?
What color a walk on the ocean's shore?
What color a chance not there before?

What color the joy of a life conceived?
A promise kept, a goal achieved?
What color the loss from heedless haste?
Of burning hate? Of needless waste?

Of joyful hearts with caring friends?
Or times of grief when friendship ends?
With eyes consigned to black of night?
What are the colors of inner sight?

Life's colors blend in patterned hues
Like light that springs from darkened muse
In soulful yearnings quest to be
The spirit's true epitome.

Yet trapped within the senses lair,
With sight as clear as mountain air,
High from a peak's commanding view,
What do you see that's not in you?

There behind the realm of sight,
There lies a greater inner light.
The colors of soul we feel inside,
Glow still in the heart of the feeble-eyed.

Deep in the black of every soul,
Hides light that makes us innately whole.
The art that grasps life's crucial key,
Holds colors of things we cannot see.

All deeper truth but lies in wait,
For inner struggle to create.
And wrestling with an artist's soul,
We seek to make the painting whole.

Much like the worm, earthbound and blind,
Our color flows from us to find,
The canvas wet until the end,
With colors we forever blend.

Where outer day meets inner night,
Where inner warmth meets outer light,
There pours from every soulful fight,
The flooding rainbow...
of inner sight.

APPENDIX

by the Editor

Having worked with Michelle for three years, I now have an opportunity to tell the story of the everyday heroics that never occurred to her as book-worthy, and yet, they document her heroism beyond survival alone and above all the horrors of her illness in the light she has sustained in its aftermath.

Michelle's involvement with life goes far beyond her high heels. A typical day begins with two specific regimes for eye-care and lung-care, and only then can she do all the things that those of us with vision could hardly imagine doing without a mirror or a light, let alone without vision, such as styling her beautiful, long hair. Her morning routine culminates in selecting her wardrobe by feeling the texture of each item of clothing, and choosing the accessories such as earrings and necklace, hoping that any matched pairs truly match each other. When she puts on her cool, fashionable high heels she feels like her former self again if only for a moment.

By the time she leaves her door she's fairly exasperated but she rises above it all, expressing her friendly personality with humor and a smile. She appears so put together she makes it look easy; but it is not. More importantly here, Michelle sustains her outward beauty only as a true reflection of her inner beauty. Not ever seeing the final result, she subconsciously honors her inner being as worthy of expression, tender care, and presentation. It is how she celebrates her soul. When she opens her arms to hug someone, it is both an act of love and an act of sacrifice. Her scars pull and contract, causing a burning sensation, but love overcomes and she does not mention it. (I just learned about this after three years and only when I asked.) While professional therapeutic massage on the scar tissue would offer relief, her health insurance does not cover it, and she remains imprisoned by internal and external scar tissue.

Obviously her everyday home life today is nothing like what it was before SJS/TEN. Everything is different. Specific voice-activated programs and other such comforts for the blind would make her life easier but have been out of reach of her budget, and with difficulty she manages without them. In all aspects of her existence she has had to adapt and adjust, and still she goes throughout her day doing the things that most of us with vision would sometimes prefer not to do: cleaning house, doing laundry, taking out the trash, answering the mail, scheduling and arranging special public transportation for appointments. She exercises at least a half hour every day on a treadmill, not to create a toned look, but to strengthen her lungs because she suffers from chronic obstructive pulmonary disease, a complication of SJS/TEN. Her concern is for preserving the percentage of lung capacity that remains, investing in the future by keeping herself up, day by day, using what she has with a sense of mindfulness and gratitude.

She carefully spends a certain amount of time in the sun every day, not to vainly work on a tan, but to take advantage of full-spectrum light which is needed by blind persons to maintain a natural circadian rhythm. She also needs the radiance of the sun to warm her body temperature as it is difficult to regulate after SJS/TEN. While in the sun she meditates, listens to audio books and music, and creates a world of peace and serenity until she is able to emanate her internal light from a condition of inner calm. Without it, she suffers.

"I am not a hero," she insisted. "I'm just a normal person trying to live my life like everyone else. My mother is the true hero."

Smiling at her natural humility, I asked Michelle if her mother's story would be her sequel. She grew silent, probably imagining three more years of intense writing. Then she smiled at the challenge. Looking upward she prayed aloud, "God give me strength!" And the spirit moved again.

Denege Patterson

Bokeelia, FL
June 2014

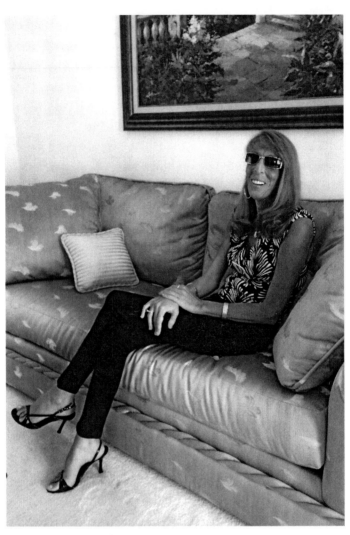

Michelle Frazzetto June 2014

ACKNOWLEDGEMENTS

by the Author

I am grateful to so many people for their support and encouragement during the writing of this book. First, thanks to my editor, Denege Patterson. Thank you for believing in my story. Without you this book would not have been possible. Through all our laughter and tears we did it! My deepest appreciation for all your help, and for sharing your knowledge and writing skills with me. In my darkest days of writing this book, you have inspired me to face my fears and encouraged me to continue. You are simply amazing, and I adore you.

Thank you to all the doctors and nurses at Greystone Hospital who took excellent care of me. To one of the most compassionate and patient persons I know, my doctor and friend, Dr. Lister. Thank you for your infinite and extraordinary dedication the last twenty-eight years.

To my doctors who worked with me after my recovery from SJS/TEN, I know as a patient I have been a medical challenge. I am grateful for all your exceptional care. Thank you, Dr. Barrow, Dr. Brueck, Dr. G. Draulans, Dr. Dunford, Dr. Flaharty, Dr. Laquis, Dr. McGrady, Dr. Palmon, Dr. Smith, Dr. Torricelli. My deepest gratitude to Dr. Dugan for your continuing care and support, and for keeping my adrenals balanced. Heartfelt thanks to my friend and Chiropractor Dr. Kelly Wallis, for coming to my home and adjusting me after a long day of writing. To Dr. Kellum, you're brilliant. 'thank you' just doesn't seem enough. To the techs and staff of Dr. Palmon's office, you girls are fantastic. Thanks for all you do.

To my Mom who prayed me back to life, my heart belongs to you. To my family: thank you. The book is finally finished! It's been a long road since SJS/TEN, but I made it! Teresa, thank God for your computer abilities; I greatly appreciate all your help. Heart-warmed thanks to my incredible friend Karen (Wa-Wa) who unrelentingly cheered me on each day, and showed her endless support. You had faith in me and motivated me through this entire book. Thank you to my wonderful friend Linda who is always in awe of me especially while I was writing this book, yet she is the remarkable one. To Daniel, thanks for all your assistance in anything I needed. You are a gem. Thank you to my friends Matthew, Patricia, Mariana, and Melanie who have taken the time out of their day to listen when I needed to decompress. To my friends who have accepted me for me and all my friends who have stood by me from the beginning, you are all true blessings. To all my "seeing-eye angels," you know who you are. I am eternally grateful. To the many friends and acquaintances who inquired and took an interest in my book, thank you. To all the people who prayed for me, thank you. Your prayers were answered.

To my editor's husband Peter, thanks for your collaboration, understanding, humor, and for sharing Denege with me the last three years. Special thanks to Sue Wild for mentioning the *News-Press* article. To Mike, thanks for the references. To reporter Amy Bennett-Williams, thank you for the most valuable piece of information. Thank you to the Peppertree family for your personal attention in accommodating me throughout the publishing process. To the parents whose children suffered through SJS/TEN, you should all be commended.

Finally, I would like to thank God for guiding me through the writing of my book, and for giving me the wisdom and strength I needed to accomplish it.

ABOUT THE AUTHOR

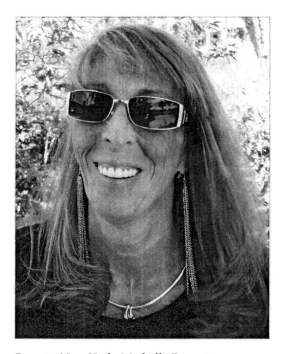

Born in New York, Michelle Frazzetto grew up speaking both Italian and English as the fourth child of first-generation Italian immigrants. Upon her graduation, she entered the world of finance in New York City. After surviving SJS/TEN, she attended a school for the blind, and college courses. She is a member of the Florida Council for the Blind, and supports the Stevens-Johnson Foundation.

www.michellefrazzetto.com

CPSIA information can be obtained at www.ICGtesting.com
Printed in the USA
BVOW04s2146291114

376860BV00001B/32/P